Conten

Introduction
Optimising Female Health

Women's 'troubles'. They're talked about a lot. In fact, they're often the subject of many a joke. But, for women who are experiencing hormonal changes, breast pain, cystitis or menstrual cramps, it's no laughing matter.

Fortunately, women have created a forum for openness about key health conditions, with everything from celebrities sharing their experiences of female cancers to health-orientated charity events bringing women's health into the open. But, while research shows that women are more likely to see a GP about their health issues than men, many also want to help manage their health conditions themselves, preferring bespoke and integrated healthcare plans that include diet, supplements, exercise, stress management and other complementary therapies.

The aim of this book is to provide you with a guide to using these therapies to optimise your overall health. After a brief introduction to the inner workings of the female body, each chapter will focus on holistic solutions for a specific female health problem. These principles are then bought together at the end of the book, where you'll find more general advice on keeping your health in tip-top condition.

As with any health condition, if you're experiencing symptoms that are particularly severe or persistent, it is important to seek advice from your doctor or health practitioner before trying to manage the condition yourself.

Chapter 1
Your Body, Your Hormones

Ask anyone what defines 'women's health' issues, and they're likely to come back with an answer that involves hormones...and they are right. But hormones aren't just there to make women tearful, temperamental and irritable! They control the whole of a woman's physiology, extending far beyond the nuts and bolts of the reproductive system. In fact, they make up an intricate biochemical system that drives how a woman thinks, feels and responds in every situation. You only need to read this book to realise just how much an influence hormones have on so many female health conditions, so let's delve a little deeper...

Powerful Regulators: Something to Consider

Hormones are, essentially, biological signallers – communicators. In order for this to happen, hormones have to be released from an endocrine gland (thyroid gland, parathyroid gland, adrenal gland or ovary, for example) and then travel through the blood system until they reach a cell with a receptor that is responsive to the shape of that particular hormone – like a lock and a key. The hormone molecule then attaches itself to the cell's receptor and sends signals inside the cell, telling it, for example, to produce a certain protein or multiply in number.

Hormones are involved in just about every biological process, including immune function, reproduction, growth and blood sugar regulation. They work in incredibly small concentrations – as low as parts per trillion, which is why hormonal disruptors, such as stress, have such a huge and wide-ranging effect (see chapter 3). But to fully appreciate the intricacies of the female hormonal cycle, it's important to first fully understand the finer points of female anatomy.

The Start of It All

From the time of birth, a girl already has in place the structures she needs to grow and change into a woman. On a basic level, this includes all the reproductive organs, both internal (vagina, uterus, fallopian tubes, ovaries) and external (labia, clitoris, hymen), as well as a full complement of eggs. During foetal life, there are about six to seven million eggs, but from this time on, no new eggs are produced. In fact, the vast majority of the eggs within the ovaries steadily die, until they are depleted at menopause. At birth, there are approximately one million eggs; and by the time of puberty, only about 300,000 remain. Of these, 300 to 400 will be ovulated during a woman's reproductive lifetime. What's interesting is that the number of eggs available is amazingly consistent from woman to woman and new tests can accurately predict a woman's fertile 'lifespan' by measuring her remaining egg stores.

Your...What-Do-You-Call-It?

We might be a little coy about the technical name, and all manner of 'avoiders' have been used to describe it, but the vagina is actually a very interesting structure. In essence, it is a fibro-muscular tube, connecting the neck of the uterus (called the cervix) with the external organs of reproduction. It runs upwards and backwards at an angle of about 45 degrees, nestled between the bladder at the front and the rectum behind. This explains why many women on their periods find they need the toilet more frequently or experience backache.

The average vagina is about 9.5cm long at its longest point and has muscular walls covered by a more delicate lining tissue. This surface is kept moist by secretions from the cervix. The cells that line the vagina also produce various compounds, which help to keep the environment inside acidic. As a result, only certain friendly bacteria, such as *Lactobacillus acidophilus*, can survive there. The purpose of this acid is to make the environment hostile to unwanted microbes (such as those from the anus), which could potentially cause infection. The downside is that it's unfavourable for sperm, which is why they swim upwards to the cervix.

Your Cervix

The cervix is a spongy opening at the top of the vagina and the entrance to the uterus (strictly speaking, it is part of the uterus itself). It is highly influenced by reproductive events, both throughout the monthly menstrual cycle and during pregnancy. Changes in the cervical mucus can indicate when a woman is fertile, while changes in the opening of the cervix can indicate how impending labour and delivery are at the end of pregnancy.

Your Uterus

The uterus is a hollow, muscular, pear-shaped organ that lies in the pelvic cavity between the urinary bladder and the rectum. It leans forward almost at right angles to the vagina, with part of its surface resting on the bladder. It stands to reason, then, that when the bladder is full, the uterus feels the pressure. The uterus is also supported by the muscles of the pelvic floor, and ligaments that suspend it from the walls of the pelvis. It's about 7.5cm long, 5cm wide and 2.5cm thick, though the thickness of the lining changes depending on the time of the month.

In total, the uterus is made up of three layers:

- The perimetrium is a tough outer layer of connective tissue that helps to keep the uterus anchored in place
- The myometrium is a thick middle layer of smooth muscle tissue, which is responsible for the contractions required during labour
- The endometrium is an inner lining layer, the top half of which is shed and renewed during the menstrual cycle

As well as being a passageway for sperm to reach the egg, the uterus is also the place where a fertilised egg can implant and grow into a baby.

Your Ovaries

The ovaries are the female 'gonads', or sex organs. Each is approximately the size and shape of an unshelled almond and attached to the upper part of uterus by a series of ligaments and bands of tissue. The ovaries themselves have two main layers of tissue, the middle part (called the medulla) is rich in blood vessels and nerves, while the outer cortex is where the ovarian follicles (eggs) grow and mature at various points during the menstrual cycle. As we'll see later, the ovaries are also the place where oestrogen and progesterone are made.

Your Fallopian Tubes

Extending from the uterus up towards the ovaries are two tubes called the fallopian tubes. Each tube is about 10cm long and provides a route for sperm to reach the egg and for the fertilised egg to travel to the uterus. The funnel-shaped portion at the end of each fallopian tube is only partially attached to the ovary. The tube itself is open ended and surrounded by finger-like projections called fimbriae, which catch the egg as it is released. Inside, the tube is lined with little hair-like structures called cilia, which help to waft the egg toward the uterus. This movement is aided by waves of muscle contraction along the tube called peristalsis.

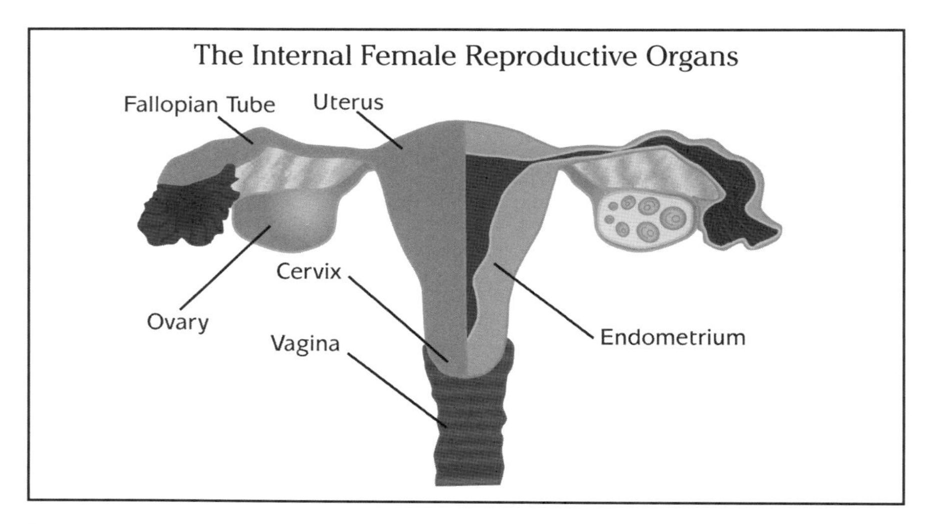

Puberty – Getting Ready for Reproduction

For about the first decade of life, the ovaries remain in an inactive state. But at around age 10, specialised endocrine glands in the brain start to release bursts of hormones that activate the start of puberty. These hormones cause the hips to widen, the breast tissue to mature and pubic hair to grow. They also trigger the onset of menstruation, which, for many females, is the most noticeable change, confirming the transition from girl to woman.

Each month, after puberty, hormones produced by the pituitary gland in the brain stimulate the maturation of an egg and initiate the regular sequence of changes in the ovaries and uterus that make up the female reproductive cycle.

The Female Reproductive Cycle

Medically speaking, each new reproductive cycle actually begins on the first day of menstrual bleeding. This first phase of the activity is aptly named the menstrual phase. In the uterus, the top layer of the endometrium is being shed, while in the brain, the anterior pituitary gland releases a substance called follicle-stimulating hormone. This causes the eggs in the ovaries to grow and mature, although usually, only one egg will mature fully enough to be ovulated.

Once a woman's period has finished, she is said to be in the pre-ovulatory phase. By this time, the cells surrounding the maturing egg have started make oestrogen. This hormone ensures that the uterus lining starts to thicken again, ready for any future pregnancy.

Around about day 12-14 of a woman's cycle, the level of oestrogen being produced by the cells around the growing egg reaches a peak. This signal is picked up by the pituitary gland, which responds by releasing a burst of a substance called luteinising hormone. This is the trigger for ovulation, causing the mature egg to be released from the ovary and begin its journey towards the uterus.

Once the egg has been released, the body enters the post-ovulatory or luteal phase. At this time of the month, the shell of cells that were surrounding the egg collapse and form a structure called the corpus luteum. This produces progesterone and small amounts of oestrogen, which prepare the body in case a pregnancy occurs. Changes that take place include a thickening of the lining of the uterus, the production of more mucus in the uterus to assist the passage of sperm to the egg and the release of cervical mucus into the vagina to help the sperm travel up into the uterus.

If no fertilisation takes place, the corpus luteum has a lifespan of just 14 days. After this time, it shrivels up and the production of progesterone and oestrogen stops. This sudden drop in hormone levels is what prompts menstrual bleeding and the start of a whole new cycle.

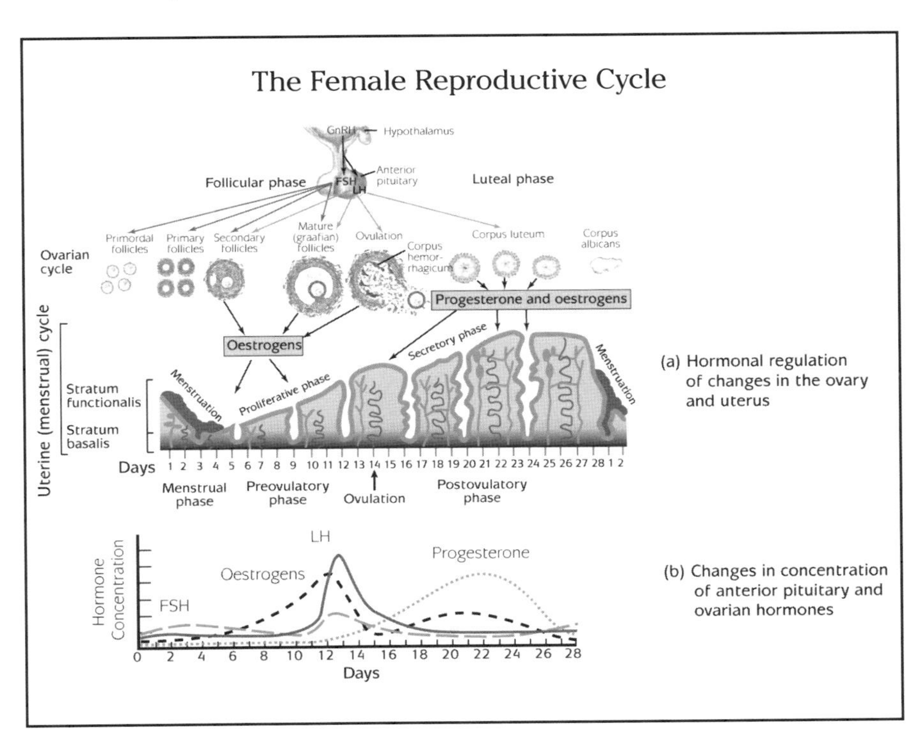

(a) Hormonal regulation of changes in the ovary and uterus

(b) Changes in concentration of anterior pituitary and ovarian hormones

Pregnancy – The Miracle of New Life

If an egg is fertilised, the events of the last part of the menstrual cycle are stalled. Rather than shrivelling up and dying, the corpus luteum lives past its normal two-week lifespan, rescued from degeneration by a hormone called human chorionic gonadotrophin (or hCG for short). This is produced by the embryo about eight days after fertilisation and stimulates the corpus luteum to keep making the hormones needed to maintain the uterine lining. It is also the hormone that is detected in pregnancy tests. About three to four months into the pregnancy, the placenta has fully developed and is able to take over this role from the corpus luteum. It produces the progesterone, oestrogen and other hormones needed for the rest of the pregnancy.

While the female hormone cycle might sound a little complicated at first glance, it does show the absolute wonder of biochemical systems. It is something that our body has prepared for during puberty, and will also down-regulate in later life.

Menopause – A Very Natural Wind-Down

The menopause isn't an 'ending', as such. It's more a 'running out' or natural wind-down. Occurring at around the age of 55, it marks the end of childbearing years and can happen slowly or suddenly, depending on each woman's own biochemistry. As a woman nears the menopause, her store of eggs becomes depleted and her body becomes less receptive to the various sex hormones.

The ovaries become less responsive to follicle-stimulating hormone and luteinising hormone, and ovulation and menstruation understandably become less predictable and ordered, until such a time as the menstrual cycle ceases. Of course, this brings with it all kinds of natural bodily responses, such as vaginal dryness (no hormones to stimulate cervical mucus release), breast shrinkage (as the body does not need to prepare for pregnancy), and sometimes, lack of sex drive. Once understood from a physiological perspective, it often reassures women that the symptoms they are experiencing are a natural occurrence, and not something peculiar.

Hormones – A Natural Approach

By understanding the biochemistry of the female hormonal system, we can understand where an appropriate eating plan, supplements, herbs and other remedies can influence women's health conditions. By reading about how different herbs and nutrients work, you will understand the logic of including them. If you want to, you can also choose to work with an experienced practitioner to assess which approach is most appropriate for you.

Chapter 2
Influencing Hormones – Your Liver and Digestive System

When considering your female sex hormones, you shouldn't just concentrate on your brain and ovaries; you should also consider the role of other body systems, such as your liver and digestive system. After all, a big part of hormonal balance relies on having effective systems in place for 'mopping up' and excreting old or excess hormones.

Introducing Your Liver

Located just under the ribs on the right-hand side of the body, the liver is your largest gland and is estimated to have over 500 functions. In order to carry out all these functions, it filters a staggering 1.4l of blood per minute. This is a mixture of oxygenated blood arriving from the heart and nutrient-enriched blood from the digestive system. These two blood supplies then mix in the liver and are processed together.

Liver Structure

The liver itself is made up of four lobes, with each lobe comprising hundreds of smaller processing units called lobules. Each lobule is made up of liver cells called hepatocytes, whose job it is to clean the blood. Overall, the structure of the liver allows substances to be taken from the bloodstream by the hepatocytes, processed and then either stored, returned to circulation for removal in the urine or deposited in the bile for excretion via the digestive system.

Liver Detoxification

One of the liver's most important functions is to break down toxins and biological substances, such as hormones. This process occurs in two steps, helpfully named phase I and phase II! These two processes can be likened to the processes of chopping up and mopping up!

In phase I, enzymes in the liver add reactive chemical groups onto the toxin to prepare for mopping up in phase II. Phase II, on the other hand, is all about reducing a toxin's reactivity and preparing for removal from the body. This is done using different biochemical reactions, each of which involves sticking a water-soluble chemical group onto the substance to create a compound that the body can safely and speedily remove. In most cases, the new chemical group reacts with the part of the toxin that was activated in the phase I reaction.

Compromised Liver Function

For healthy detoxification, it's important that the phase I and II liver pathways function in balance. If toxins are chopped up faster than they can be mopped up, the reactive intermediates that result from phase I can build up in the liver. What's more, imbalanced liver function leads to changes in metabolism that can affect the body's ability to handle toxins, as well as influencing the levels of various hormones in the body.

Hormones and Your Liver

Just like drugs, toxins and other unwanted biochemical substances, sex hormones are metabolised both by phase I and phase II of the liver's processes. Proper liver function is therefore vital for healthy hormonal balance.

When looking at hormone detoxification, the liver's role in oestrogen metabolism is usually considered to be more important than the process of progesterone metabolism. This is partly because progesterone has a multi-pathway metabolism (allowing it to be converted into other useful hormones instead of having to be processed through the liver), and partly because, compared to other hormones, relatively small amounts of oestrogen are required to have an action in the body. This means that proper control mechanisms to balance the level of oestrogen are even more important than for other biochemicals.

Oestrogen

When oestrogen is released into the bloodstream, the majority of it is attached to a carrier molecule called sex-hormone-binding globulin. This is a kind of hormone-carrying taxi that is made by the liver to help keep the level of 'free oestrogen' (and testosterone) in the bloodstream in check. Adequate production of sex-hormone-binding globulin is therefore vital to ensure there isn't too much free oestrogen running around the body.

Once free oestrogen has engaged with its receptor and sent a message into a cell, it's important that it is quickly inactivated and excreted. If oestrogen is allowed to build up in the body, its delicate ebb and flow becomes disturbed and hormonal imbalances can result. This inactivation and excretion is carried out by the liver.

During phase I of liver detoxification, oestrogen can be turned into one of three different substances. Since these substances are all reactive, potentially damaging molecules, they need to be quickly mopped up by the liver phase II processes. These phase II processes are sometimes referred to as 'conjugation reactions' (conjugation means 'formed by the union of two substances') and simply involves attaching the reactive oestrogen to a chemical group that makes it less harmful and more water-soluble. This means the oestrogen can then be deposited in the bile or bloodstream ready for excretion via the digestive tract or urine.

Supporting Your Liver

It makes sense that, as your hormones are metabolised and eventually pass through your liver on their way out of the body, an overloaded liver will struggle to keep up with demand. This is why many natural healthcare practitioners will consider the health of your liver if you are having hormonal problems.

Signs and symptoms to look out for, which indicate your liver may not be functioning at its best, include:

- Poor appetite or nausea, especially in the morning
- Difficulty digesting fatty foods
- Gallstones
- Pale, fatty stools that float
- Constipation
- Intolerance to alcohol
- Dry skin
- Skin rashes
- Itching on the arms, legs, palms of the hands and soles of the feet
- Tiredness and fatigue
- Problems sleeping, typically waking between 1am and 3am
- Slight yellowing of the whites of eyes
- Dark circles under the eyes
- High cholesterol levels
- Hormone imbalances
- A weakened immune system
- Weight gain, especially around the abdomen
- Cellulite
- Excessive sweating
- Offensive body odour
- A feeling of overheating

- Mood changes, such as anger and irritability
- Poor concentration
- Brain fog
- Recurrent headaches
- Multiple allergies and sensitivities

If these symptoms sound all too familiar, it's advisable to start supporting your liver with the seven-day detox programme below and some liver-supporting nutrients.

Seven-Day Detox Plan

During the seven-day cleanse, you still need to eat regularly, but keep meals simple and nourishing. Eat plenty of organic vegetables, wholegrains and fruit with small amounts of light organic protein, such as chicken, fish and pulses.

It's also important to drink at least 2l of fluids, such as filtered water, raw vegetable juices and herbal teas each day to prevent constipation and help your kidneys to eliminate the toxins that the liver has broken down.

Key foods to avoid during the cleanse are dairy products, fried foods, refined foods, sugar and sweets, fizzy drinks, cakes and biscuits, and anything made with artificial sweeteners and colourings, flavourings and preservatives. You also need to cut out all black tea, coffee, caffeinated drinks and alcohol, to give your liver a break, so it can throw off any toxins.

For the seven days of the cleanse, you need to take the following liver flush drink first thing in the morning, before you eat or drink anything.

In a liquidiser, mix together the following, blend until smooth and then drink slowly.

200ml fresh lemon juice
200ml spring water or mineral water
1 clove fresh garlic
1tbsp organic cold pressed flax seed oil
1cm finely grated root ginger
1 pinch cayenne pepper

During the cleanse, you may find you experience skin flare-ups, headaches, flu-like symptoms or unusual emotions. These are a positive indication that your body is detoxifying.

Once your seven-day detox is over, taking a combination of liver-supporting nutrients and following the principles laid out in chapter 15 will help to keep your liver functioning at its best.

Nutrients for Liver Support

Nutrients recommended for liver function, which specifically relate to hormonal balance, include:

- B vitamins – these support phase I processes in the liver and help the liver to successfully form oestrogen conjugates
- Antioxidants – these are nutrients that destroy free radicals and so help protect the liver cells from harmful phase I metabolites. The most important antioxidants for the liver are vitamin C, vitamin E and alpha lipoic acid
- N-acetyl-cysteine – this is a sulphur-based amino acid that is important for one of the liver's main detoxification pathways. It is also needed to make glutathione, a potent antioxidant that is produced in the liver, where it helps to protect the liver from damage by phase I intermediates
- Choline, inositol and methionine – these liver-protective nutrients are important for ferrying fat through the liver and methionine, in particular, is used by the liver to deactivate excess oestrogen
- Taurine – as a sulphur-containing amino acid, taurine supports the phase II sulphation pathway, which is one of the pathways used to metabolise oestrogen. Taurine also stimulates bile production and excretion, aiding the elimination of the liver's waste products through the digestive system
- Glutamine – this is needed for the proper function of one of the liver's detoxification pathways. It can be used by the liver to make extra supplies of the antioxidant glutathione

For a more long-term liver support, it's best to take a combination of these nutrients twice a day with meals for two to three months.

Hormone Recycling and Your Digestive Tract

Your digestive system also plays an important role in the balancing of hormones within the body. This is because hormone conjugates are excreted from the liver through the bilary tract. Put simply, this is the pathway of pipes that carries bile from the liver to the gallbladder (where the bile is stored and concentrated) and then out to the intestine.

The primary purpose of bile is to help the body digest fats properly, but it also serves as a useful vehicle for getting rid of waste products by depositing them in the digestive tract, where they can be eliminated with the faeces. However, in order for this to work effectively, it's important that the waste product stays attached to the chemical group that was added in phase II liver metabolism. If this is removed, the toxins can be reabsorbed, creating extra work for the liver!

One of the chemical 'conjugates' added to oestrogen in phase II is a substance called glucuronic acid. Unfortunately, certain types of bacteria that live in the gut can produce a substance called beta-glucuronidase, which can break the glucuronic acid off the oestrogen molecule, allowing it to be reabsorbed. This most commonly occurs when the gut transit time is slower than normal. This can be the result of poor digestion, constipation due to a lack of bulky fibrous matter in the diet or stress (which can slow the digestive system down). It's also been shown that diets high in heavy protein and saturated fat can increase the levels of beta-glucuronidase made in the gut.

Research on women with different diets has shown that vegetarian women with higher fibre intakes have higher levels of oestrogen breakdown products in the faeces, indicating good clearance, while women on meat-eating diets (high fat and protein and low dietary fibre) had higher levels of plasma (blood) oestrogen, showing poorer clearance in the liver. This is why, for overall hormonal health, it's important to ensure you're getting plenty of fibre in your diet (see chapter 15) and that your bowels are moving at least once a day. Supplementing with friendly bacteria can also help to maintain overall healthy digestive balance and favourably affect gut transit time.

- A good probiotic regime should include one capsule of high-potency probiotic with water before each meal. This should be a high-strength supplement containing a mixture of friendly *Lactobacilli* and *Bifidobacteria* strains that are resistant to stomach acid and bile. This ensures the bacteria reach the intestines alive.

If, after following the dietary principles in chapter 15, you still find that your digestion is on the sluggish side, you might find it useful to include a colon-cleansing supplement containing a gentle form of fibre, such as flax, along with digestive herbs, such as fennel, clove, fenugreek and liquorice, and a probiotic.

Taking the Pill? Consider Your Liver

When people talk about 'the pill', they're usually referring to the combined oral contraceptive pill, which contains synthetic versions of the hormones oestrogen and progesterone. Taken daily, for 21 days of the month, the relatively high levels of hormones in the pill override the natural hormonal balance and inhibit egg development in the ovaries. This, in turn, prevents the luteinising hormone surge, which usually triggers ovulation.

It is a highly effective form of contraception for many women, but some natural practitioners have reservations about the widespread use of the pill. This is because the extra hormones in the pill create a lot of extra work for the liver and can cause the body to use up certain nutrients, such as B vitamins, vitamin C, magnesium and zinc, more quickly. There are also concerns that the hormones in the pill, which are excreted through the bowels and urinary system, are ending up in lakes, rivers and the water supply.

If you're thinking of trying for a baby, health advisors suggest that you wait for between one and three months after coming off the pill before trying to conceive, to give your body a chance to adapt back to its own hormonal cycles before embarking on the hormonally turbulent experience of pregnancy. The amount of time that it takes to clear the pill from your system depends on many factors; your age, how long you were on the pill, what kind of pill you were on, your general health and of course the health of your liver and digestive system.

Waiting a few months also allows you to more accurately date a pregnancy, and means that you can put into place a healthy pregnancy regime, such as taking folic acid and cutting back on smoking and alcohol, before the event actually takes place. At this time, some women choose to follow a liver detox programme, which will encourage healthy liver function, including clearance of the pill from the body.

Chapter 3
Influencing Hormones – Sugar Balance and Stress

Blood sugar balance and stress – these are two factors which go hand in hand, and which greatly affect hormonal balance, yet often go untempered in women with other hormonal disturbances. However, getting these right will have a powerfully positive effect on your hormonal well-being.

Blood Sugar Balance

You might have heard it said that taking on a large amount of dietary sugar in one go (a sugar 'hit', from foods such as chocolate, for example) can cause a massive insulin response in the body, which can then result in a blood sugar crash.

After you eat, sweet and starchy foods are broken down into glucose, a simple sugar that is the main source of energy for the body's cells. However, in order to keep the body healthy, this sugar can't be allowed to just run around freely. Instead, a hormone called insulin, which is made by the pancreas, tightly controls the level of sugar in the blood.

Insulin has become widely known because of the condition diabetes, but many people don't appreciate how finely tuned and powerful this wonderful hormone is, encouraging the uptake of glucose by body cells, and the storage of extra glucose by the body as glycogen (in the muscles and liver) and as fat.

So What's Going Wrong?

Most of the time, this system works efficiently, but it's likely that, at some point, you've also experienced a 'sugar rush'. This happens when a massive load of sugar enters the bloodstream in one go, causing the body to respond by releasing a larger than normal release of insulin. If this insulin release overshoots the mark, the blood sugar can swing too low.

If this occurs on an occasional basis, the body is well tuned enough to avoid the ill effects of such dramatic sugar level changes, and, for most people, blood sugar balance is well regulated. However, many Western diets are overloaded with sugary foods and refined carbohydrates, causing a constant flux in insulin levels.

These constant sugar highs and lows can cause physiological upset, resulting in irritability, a fluttering feeling in the chest, anxiety, nervous tension, sweating, dizziness, restlessness, headache, lack of concentration, fatigue, craving for sweet foods, lack of appetite or constant hunger, depression and being unusually emotional. These are all symptoms that are remarkably similar to the symptoms of PMS!

From a health perspective, someone presenting with symptoms of irritability, anxiety, nervous tension, sweating, restlessness, headaches and food cravings might ordinarily be assumed to have a hormonal imbalance. In these cases, working to rebalance blood sugar levels, as well as addressing stress levels, can have an effect on all hormonal symptoms.

The Link to Stress

In an intricately and finely tuned mingling of biochemical systems, stress influences blood sugar, and this can have very real effects on your hormonal system in ways that most women haven't even heard about.

Research has shown that stress itself leads to an increase in blood sugar. This is because when you're stressed, the body releases 'fight or flight' hormones, such as adrenalin and cortisol, one of the functions of which is to raise blood sugar levels to help with either combating, or running away. Although this makes perfect physiological sense, when you think how many times a day you feel threatened, anxious or on edge, you can easily see how much of an impact increased stress levels can have on blood sugar balance. In fact, studies have shown that even perceived stress can elicit a cortisol release and impact on blood sugar levels.

As well as influencing the blood sugar level, cortisol's effects include a burst of energy, heightened memory and lowered sensitivity to pain. All this sounds great, and it is when it only happens now and then, and when the body's relaxation response, which includes a down-regulation of cortisol, insulin and other hormones involved in heart rate and blood pressure, freely occurs to bring about a state of physiological normality. But here's the dilemma. Many women are living incredibly stressful, anxious lives. Instead of regularly entering relaxation response, their stressed state is maintained. Over time, prolonged release of cortisol in the body can lead to negative effects, such as impaired cognitive performance, suppressed thyroid function, high blood pressure, decreased immunity and blood sugar imbalances. It can also have knock-on effects on other hormones.

The Pregnenolone Steal...

In chronic stress situations, the constant need for cortisol by the body can start to impact on the manufacture of other hormones. This is because both the sex hormones and cortisol are made from the same precursor, a substance called pregnenolone.

Pregnenolone has two main fates. It can be converted into progesterone and then on into other adrenal hormones, such as cortisol when a stress response is needed, and it can also be converted into the hormone DHEA, from which oestrogen is made.

The problem is that these pathways are not always serviced equally. For example, in prolonged stressful situations, the body's demand for cortisol (and other adrenal hormones) is high. As a result, the body uses pregnenolone predominantly to support the production of stress hormones, at the expense of making progesterone, DHEA and oestrogen. This can have all kinds of knock-on effects on hormonal balance, resulting in restlessness, irritability, sweating, lack of libido, unpredictable hormonal cycles and unusual emotional symptoms.

The Solution?

To support hormonal balance in a truly holistic way, it's vital not only to control blood sugar balance, but also to help to manage stress.

STEP ONE: Balance Your Blood Sugar Levels Through Diet

Basing your food choices on regular portions of lean protein with complex carbohydrates, such as those found in vegetables and wholegrains, is an excellent way to naturally support blood sugar and hormonal balance. By following a low-glycaemic diet, rather than eating lots of refined and sugary carbohydrates (which raise blood glucose and insulin levels quickly), you will not only benefit from more stable eating patterns, but you might also lose excess weight. This again helps to stabilise hormones, especially if oestrogen dominance is a problem. What's more, wholefood diets rich in vegetables, wholegrains, beans and pulses are also rich in many of the nutrients which help hormonal balance, especially B vitamins and important hormone-influencing minerals, such as magnesium, zinc and manganese. For more information on what to eat to balance your blood sugar levels, see chapter 15.

STEP TWO: Manage Your Sweet Craving Triggers

To help you on the road to better blood sugar balance, it's also important to learn to manage sugar cravings. The good news is that low-glycaemic foods keep you feeling fuller for longer and so should help to curb a sweet tooth, but we're all human and food association is a powerful thing! What we hear, see and learn all conditions what we feel about food. Here are just a few of the perceptions that you might have to master, when it comes to your favourite sugar snacks:

"I'm premenstrual; something sweet will make me feel better."
"I'm stressed out; I need something sweet to give me a lift."
"I'm tired, I'm angry, I'm bored; I need sweet food."
"I'm having a coffee; time for some sweet food."
"I've had a good meal...bring out the dessert."

We're all shaped by food association; the key is to be aware of these perceptions and recognise that your body's actual needs may be different to what you're perceiving at the time. Sometimes, the desire for sweet food is purely habit. At other times, it can represent a different unmet need, such as a need to sleep when tired or wanting take some time out when under pressure. In some cases, sweet cravings are actually triggered by a need for more fuel. This is common during menstruation, when a woman actually needs around 200 extra kcals to support her body while she bleeds. The key is to provide the body with regular low-GI meals and snacks to reduce the need to reach for something sugary. In addition, there are also a couple of supplements that can really help with the cravings.

- Glutamine is an amino acid that has a balancing effect on blood sugar levels. On the one hand, it can be used by the body to make glucose when blood sugar levels dip too low; on the other, it can help your cells respond to insulin more effectively, aiding in the management of high blood sugar levels. To curb cravings, put one to two heaped teaspoons of glutamine powder in a large bottle of water and sip through the day.

- Chromium is an essential mineral that has similar blood-sugar-balancing effects to glutamine, but works in a slightly different way. It helps ensure cells remain sensitive to insulin, which, in turn, helps to balance the level of sugar in the bloodstream. This has the added benefit of helping to keep sugar cravings at bay. For mild symptoms, 200mcg of chromium in either the GTF (glucose tolerance factor) or picolinate form per day is normally sufficient, but this dose can be increased to 200mcg, three times a day, if your cravings are severe.

STEP THREE: Manage Stress

Easy to say, but not so easy to do! You may find incorporating some of the suggestions in chapter 16 and 17 are of benefit. Alternatively, if your stress levels are very high, you might prefer to talk to a specialist practitioner who can help you address your stress in a more personalised way.

Chapter 4
Premenstrual Syndrome: PMS

PMS is talked about, joked about, lived with and put up with. Women around the world suffer its effects in varying degrees every month. From simple irritability through to serious mood swings and emotional unpredictability, PMS needs to be understood and properly managed.

What is PMS?

PMS is disorder that occurs in the luteal phase of the menstrual cycle (see chapter 1) in the two weeks leading up to menstruation. It can affect a woman at any stage of her reproductive life, including the teens and twenties; however, it does seem to peak in women aged between 30 and 40.

PMS produces a wide range of physical and emotional changes, including bloating, backache, breast tenderness, food cravings, fatigue, irritability and, sometimes, depression. It generally occurs consistently and predictably from month to month and women can suffer few or many symptoms, which can be so severe they interfere with everyday life. Keeping a diary and monitoring your symptoms in order to gauge a pattern will help you to decide if you are suffering from PMS.

Symptoms of PMS

Physiological	**Psychological**
Bloating	Irritability
Weight gain	Tension
Breast tenderness	Anxiety
Headache/Migraine	Mood swings
Pelvic discomfort and pain	Aggression
Change in bowel habits	Loss of concentration
Increase in appetite	Depression
Sugar cravings	Forgetfulness
Physical tiredness	Mental tiredness

Weakness	Insomnia
Clumsiness	Change in libido
General aches and pains	Crying spells

The direct cause of PMS is not exactly known, but there are a number of factors that are thought to play a role, including hormonal and biological imbalances, nutritional insufficiencies and psychological factors.

Hormone Imbalances

As with most 'monthly-cycle'-related conditions, it stands to reason that hormonal status can affect your chance of getting PMS. Scientists have, for many years, thought that increased oestrogen is the main cause of PMS, and results either from increased baseline oestrogen levels, or from a lack of progesterone secretion by the corpus luteum. But there are other theories as well. As we have seen in chapter 2, clearance of oestrogen by the liver and the gut are also vital in maintaining oestrogen balance.

Though PMS symptoms are most often linked with oestrogen excess, there are some cases where progesterone excess might be a factor instead. One cause of this type of imbalance could be the use and slowed excretion of synthetic progestins. These are progesterone-like drugs found in hormonal medications, such as the pill. Another possible cause is a relative excess of progesterone, due to falling levels of oestrogen in the run-up to a woman's period. This has been noted in PMS sufferers who experience depression.

Nutrient Deficiencies

B vitamin insufficiencies, especially vitamin B6, as well as low levels of magnesium, can decrease the liver's ability to successfully detoxify oestrogen. This might explain why some women with severe PMS have improved symptoms when taking complexes containing these nutrients.

Blood Sugar Imbalances

Other research has linked PMS to a state of low blood sugar, with studies showing that women with PMS are more likely to experience a significant drop in blood sugar after eating, accompanied by edginess and irritability. As we saw in chapter three, blood sugar dips can trigger symptoms such as tetchiness, anxiety, cravings for sweet foods and low mood, so working with a diet and supplements to keep your blood sugar levels balanced is especially important if you suffer with PMS.

Suppressed Dopamine Levels

Anyone who has experienced PMS will know that mood can be greatly affected. Naturopathic research in the United States in the 1990s showed that oestrogens can suppress the action of dopamine, a neurotransmitter that helps to create the feeling of relaxation and mental alertness. Dopamine also affects the adrenal glands and the kidneys, which could explain why some women experience premenstrual water retention. Interestingly, vitamin B6, vitamin C and magnesium, as well as a good supply of the amino acid tyrosine, are all required for production of dopamine.

Low Serotonin Levels

Serotonin is a neurotransmitter involved in regulating mood, appetite, the sleep-wake cycle and various other bodily functions. Research has shown that low levels of serotonin are present in women suffering from premenstrual dysphoric disorder (PMDD), a severe form of PMS. It's also been suggested that women who suffer with mood swings, depression, anxiety or food cravings, or have trouble sleeping, during PMS, could also be affected. This theory is supported by laboratory findings, which show that oestrogen prevents serotonin from breaking down. Since oestrogen levels are at their lowest in the run-up to menstruation, it's possible that a woman's dropping oestrogen levels may lead to a parallel drop in serotonin.

Excess Prolactin

Some women with PMS have abnormally elevated amounts of a pituitary hormone called prolactin. Prolactin is naturally produced during breastfeeding, but levels can also increase with stress (because stress depletes dopamine, and dopamine keeps prolactin in check!) Elevated levels of prolactin can cause menstrual abnormalities and are thought to be responsible for some PMS symptoms, including breast tenderness and swelling, anxiety and irritability. This is because prolactin decreases the life of the corpus luteum, which, in turn, affects the balance between progesterone and oestrogen. In addition to the effects of stress on prolactin, excess oestrogen levels, an underactive thyroid, dopamine deficiency and a lack of vitamins B6, B3 and C, as well as zinc and magnesium, can all lead to higher-than-normal prolactin levels. In addition, diets high in saturated fat or protein are also thought to increase secretion of prolactin.

Prostaglandins

Prostaglandins are hormone-like chemicals that are made from fatty acids. They have a number of different roles in the body, including promoting smooth muscle contraction, helping to dilate blood vessels and balancing inflammation.

But research has shown that women with PMS make less anti-inflammatory prostaglandins in the luteal phase of their cycle compared to non-PMS sufferers. This lack of inflammation-dampening messengers is thought to be one of the factors responsible for the symptoms of PMS that actually cause physical pain, such as cramps, backaches, breast tenderness and headaches.

Lots of different factors can influence the balance of prostaglandins and, therefore, inflammation. Positive influences include a healthy balanced intake of essential fatty acids and optimal intake of the nutrients magnesium, vitamin B6, vitamin B3, zinc and vitamin C. Negative factors, on the other hand, are diets high in saturated fat and refined sugars, plus alcohol and stress.

Endorphins – Pain Controllers...and Much More

Endorphins are neuropeptide hormones, which are not only involved with pain management, but also help to manage appetite and emotions. Because PMS involves many physiological symptoms, including pain, it's been suggested that a change in the ratio of progesterone to oestrogen in the week or so leading up to menstruation can bring changes in endorphin activity, causing disturbances in mood, behaviour and pain perception.

Managing PMS

It's clear from the above that there are many different nutrients and dietary factors than can influence PMS. The good news is that most of these can be accounted for by following the advice in the hormone-balancing diet (see chapter 15) and taking a multinutrient specially designed for the premenstrual part of your cycle.

- A good PMS complex will contain optimal levels of B vitamins, especially B3 and B6, along with vitamin C, magnesium, zinc and chromium. Also look out for herbs, such as fennel, dandelion, American ginseng and hop flowers, which support the digestion, liver, adrenals (stress glands) and nervous system respectively.

However, there are other supplements that you should consider, which can be added to your programme to make it more specific to your personal symptoms.

Agnus Castus

Agnus castus is highly popular for PMS symptoms such as cramp, depression, mood swings, water retention and weight gain. It acts on the pituitary gland to stimulate secretion of luteinising hormone, which, in turn, stimulates the secretion of progesterone and therefore helps balance high oestrogen levels. It also inhibits the secretion of prolactin from the pituitary gland, which can help reduce symptoms such as breast tenderness.

- The recommended dose of agnus castus is 4mg of extract (equivalent to 28-52mg of agnus castus).

Vitamin E

Vitamin E has been shown to be of benefit to women experiencing PMS, especially breast symptoms.

- A good dose is 124mg of a natural, easy-to-absorb form of vitamin E, two to three times a day for a period of at least 12 weeks.

Starflower Oil

Starflower oil contains gamma-linolenic acid (GLA), which is a precursor for the production of a family of anti-inflammatory prostaglandins that regulate sex hormones and also influence inflammatory reactions. Some women with PMS struggle to make enough GLA, which can cause them to become abnormally sensitive to prolactin. This then leads to symptoms such as breast tenderness, water retention and mood changes. Consequently, women treated with GLA have shown improvements in breast pain, fluid retention and depression.

- An effective dose is one 1000mg capsule daily.

Omega 3

With most inflammatory conditions, practitioners will suggest omega 3 essential fatty acids, such as EPA and DHA from fish oil or alpha linolenic acid from flax seed oil. This is because these fats can positively influence the action of prostaglandins in the body – downscaling unwanted inflammatory responses.

- To benefit from this effect, take two to three 1000mg capsules of either a high-purity omega 3 fish oil, or flax seed oil, each day.

Phytoestrogens

Phytoestrogens are substances similar in structure to oestrogens that occur naturally in plants. They have a modulating effect on our hormones and remarkably, can help us when our hormone levels are too low, but also if levels are too high. They have become highly popular in managing many hormonal imbalances in women – not just for the menopause (when oestrogen levels become low) but also for PMS, when oestrogen levels can be imbalanced.

We already know that many body cells have oestrogen receptors, which the oestrogen locks onto to elicit its biological effects. So, when natural oestrogen levels are low, phytoestrogens can lock onto the oestrogen receptors and give a positive, though mild, oestrogenic effect. When oestrogen levels in the body are high, they can lock into oestrogen receptor sites – again, giving a weakly oestrogenic effect, which acts to downscale the overall oestrogen activity in the body. Clever!

There will be some phytoestrogens in almost all fruit, vegetables and cereals, but the food with the highest level of natural phytoestrogens is soya. This is naturally rich in phytoestrogenic compounds called isoflavones. In Japan and other Eastern countries, soy is traditionally eaten in the form of fermented whole foods, such as miso, tempeh and natto. This fermentation converts the phytoestrogenic isoflavones into their absorbable and active form, making them much more effective. However, many people find these traditional forms of soy unpalatable or difficult to obtain. A good alternative is fully fermented, wholefood soy tablets, which provide a therapeutic dose of activated isoflavones in the natural, supportive soy matrix.

- For best results, take one 1000mg tablet of high-potency, fermentation-activated whole soya, providing a total of 40mg isoflavones per tablet, each day.

Managing Mood

There are also a number of nutrients that can help to take the edge off the mood changes many women experience before their period. These include:

- 5HTP – this is used by the body to create serotonin and can therefore be very useful for PMS symptoms associated with low serotonin levels, such as depression, poor sleep and food cravings. The recommended dose is 50-100mg a day. 5HTP is best taken in a complex that also contains B vitamins and zinc, which help its conversion to serotonin.
- Tyrosine – this amino acid is needed by the body to make the pleasure and motivation neurotransmitter dopamine. A good dose is 400-500mg per day away from food in a complex that also contains B vitamins.
- Taurine – this is an amino acid that supports feelings of calm. It has a similar chemical structure to the brain's natural calming neurotransmitter, GABA, so it can provide a similar anti-anxiety effect. Taurine also reduces the release of the hormone adrenaline, protecting you from the adverse effects of stress. The recommended dose of taurine is 500-600mg twice daily. Like tyrosine, this is best taken in between meals as part of a complex containing B vitamins.
- L-theanine – this amino acid is naturally found in green tea and helps to promote relaxation by increasing alpha brainwave activity. It can also increase the level of serotonin and dopamine, providing additional mood benefits and aiding restful sleep. The optimum dose is 50-100mg per day.

- Lemon balm (*Melissa officinalis*) – this calming herb is a member of the mint family. It was used as far back as the Middle Ages to reduce stress and anxiety and promote sleep.
- Passion flower – this is a gentle yet effective relaxing agent that can be used any time of the day or night. It acts on GABA receptors in the brain and can help to calm racing thoughts and promote restful sleep.
- St Johns wort – traditionally used to support low mood, St John's wort has been shown to reduce the breakdown and re-uptake of serotonin and dopamine. Other studies have shown that St John's wort can bind to GABA receptors, as well as causing changes in signalling process in the body, which lead to reduced excitability and improved mood. More recently, scientists have also found evidence that this amazing herb might also help regulate the body's stress response. However, there is one downside! St John's wort can't be taken alongside a lot of medications, including the contraceptive pill, so if you're taking any medications, make sure you read the pack carefully or seek advice. If St John's wort is suitable for you, then a good dose is one tablet per day containing 425mg of St John's wort extract.

With so many different supplements to choose from, you might be starting to feel anxious and stressed just trying to decide which ones to take, but don't despair! If one particular nutrient or herb isn't jumping out at you, then the easiest solution is to opt for a complex.

- If your symptoms are predominated by feeling depressed, then look for a complex designed to support a positive mood, containing 5HTP, tyrosine, B vitamins, lemon balm and other beneficial nutrients.

- On the other hand, if you suffer more with feelings of anxiety and tension, go for a complex aimed at supporting the nervous system. This will contain nutrients such as taurine, B vitamins, magnesium, theanine, lemon balm and passion flower.

Chapter 5
Polycystic Ovarian Syndrome

Polycystic ovary syndrome (PCOS) is a complex condition that affects the ovaries. Typically, with PCOS, the ovaries are larger than normal and the outer surface of the ovary is covered with lots of abnormal small follicles.

What is Polycystic Ovarian Syndrome?

As the name suggests, the ovaries are polycystic. The 'cysts' themselves are actually small and immature follicles (developing eggs), but they rarely, if ever, develop fully or become ovulated. If they're not released, these small follicles continue to grow as cysts on the ovary and progesterone is not made. If released and fertilised, the follicle's relative immaturity means that a long-term pregnancy rarely results. In fact, of all women who are having trouble conceiving due to ovulation problems, 75% are thought to have PCOS to some extent. Not surprisingly, ovaries that have multiple follicles with multiple cysts will cause the sufferer a hormonal imbalance, which can lead to an array of symptoms.

Symptoms of PCOS

- Oligomenorrhoea (infrequent periods) – this can vary from a regular but elongated cycle with periods every six weeks or so, through to irregular periods occurring just once or twice a year
- Hirsutism (excess hair growth) – usually found under the chin, or on the upper lip, excess hair can also appear on the forearms, lower legs and in a line running down from the navel on the abdomen
- Acne – this usually on the face, typically appearing on the jaw line
- Infertility – this is a common consequence of the infrequent or absent ovulation that occurs in PCOS
- Miscarriage – this is more common in PCOS sufferers due to the raised level of luteinising hormone. Women with raised levels of this hormone have a 65% miscarriage rate, compared to those with normal levels (12% miscarriage rate)

- Obesity – women with PCOS often have insulin resistance, a condition in which the cells in the body are less responsive to insulin. This makes it more difficult for the body to direct glucose in the cells and causes the body to store more sugars as fat

Understanding the Hormonal Causes

Research over the years has identified various hormonal disturbances in women with PCOS. In fact, hormonal upset will be noted in 50% of women presenting with this condition.

With PCOS, there are notable increases in the levels of luteinising hormone, particularly in the very early part of the menstrual cycle, causing blood levels to become raised. This is accompanied by an increase in the level of the male hormone, testosterone, produced by the ovaries. While women naturally have inherent levels of male hormones in the body (usually having very subtle physiological effects), the greatly elevated levels in PCOS sufferers results in the facial acne, excess body hair and male pattern baldness. This hormonal imbalance is compounded by the fact that women with PCOS typically make reduced levels of sex-hormone-binding globulin – an important carrier protein that helps to keep the levels of circulating sex hormones under control (see chapter 2).

Another feature of PCOS is an increase in the level of circulating insulin and resistance to its actions. As a result, women with PCOS often gain weight around the middle and may experience cravings for carbohydrates and sugary foods. In addition to this, insulin resistance also encourages the ovaries to make more male hormones and increases the chance of developing cardiovascular disease and diabetes.

Another hormone of interest is prolactin. Compared to women with normal menstrual cycles, women with PCOS tend to have higher levels of prolactin. This not only suppresses ovulation and interferes with the menstrual cycle, but it can also lead to symptoms such as fluid retention, breast tenderness and loss of libido.

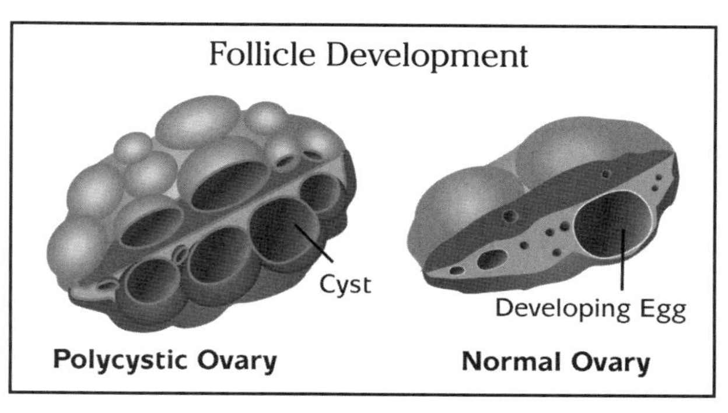

Is PCOS in Your Genes?

Interestingly, there is also a genetic basis for PCOS that has been traced back to several different genes. This explains why there are so many different severities and expressions of symptoms. For example, research shows that PCOS is more likely to be passed on if there is a family history of type II diabetes. There are also studies that show a link between early baldness (before the age of 30) in the male relatives in the woman's family and increased risk of PCOS. Women are also more at risk if they are overweight or obese, as this can result in hormonal abnormalities that can further inhibit ovulation.

Nutritional Approaches to PCOS

Manage Your Weight

We've already seen that a high percentage of women with PCOS are overweight and that this is linked in with insulin resistance. However, it is also important to understand that being overweight can actually exacerbate insulin resistance and worsen the other hormonal imbalances in PCOS. For this reason, it is really is important to adopt a diet that will help you achieve your ideal body weight and balance your insulin levels. Studies have shown that weight loss can help normalise the fertility problems associated with PCOS, reduce the levels of male hormones being produced and reduce the risk of PCOS-associated diseases.

Since PCOS is linked to insulin resistance, a low-carbohydrate diet has been shown to be one of the most successful models for aiding weight loss and reducing insulin levels. But this doesn't mean adopting an old-fashioned style Atkins' diet packed with meat, cheese and eggs! Instead, you need to eat plenty of vegetables and moderate amounts of lean protein (chicken, fish, eggs, etc), fruits, nuts, seeds and legumes to provide your body with a good supply of healthy fats, B vitamins, vitamin C and important hormone-influencing minerals, such as magnesium, zinc and manganese.

This means eliminating (or at least greatly limiting your consumption of) the following grains and all products made from them, as well as excluding all refined and sugary foods.

- Amaranth
- Barley, including barley malt
- Bran
- Buckwheat
- Bulgur
- Corn
- Cornflour
- Cornmeal

- Couscous
- Farina
- Kamut
- Millet
- Oats
- Orzo
- Quinoa
- Rice
- Rye
- Semolina
- Spelt
- Wheat

This balanced version of a low-carbohydrate diet helps to reduce excess insulin, decrease inflammation and encourage weight loss, all of which are beneficial for women with PCOS.

Meal Ideas for a Healthy, Low-Carbohydrate Diet

Breakfast

2 poached organic eggs, served with grilled mushrooms and tomatoes
Spinach omelette made with 2 organic eggs
Scrambled tofu with grilled mushrooms and tomatoes
Vegetable frittata
A smoothie made with hemp protein, almond milk, berries and pumpkin seed butter
A bowl of berries topped with plain live yoghurt (or soya yoghurt), topped with mixed seeds
Low-fat cottage cheese with berries and a sprinkle of seeds

Lunch

Greek salad with extra protein added, such as hard-boiled eggs, chicken or seafood
Chicken salad with added sugar snap peas, chopped red pepper and walnuts
Tuna salad with greens, tomato and avocado
Chicken, avocado and chickpea salad
Mixed bean salad served with green salad leaves
Lentil soup with vegetable sticks
Hummus with vegetable sticks, olives and flax seed crackers

Dinner

Grilled or baked fish topped with ratatouille, served with steamed broccoli and courgettes

Prawn curry with ground almonds, served with red cabbage and cauliflower

Grilled chicken and roasted Mediterranean vegetables

Grilled tuna with spice rub, served with mixed vegetable skewers

Stir-fried organic chicken, prawns, tempeh or tofu with peppers, mushroom, shredded cabbage, broccoli etc

Chilli made with mixed beans, served with vegetables or salad and large Romaine lettuce leaves to use as tacos!

Chickpea curry served with 3 different coloured vegetables

Salmon niçoise salad with butter beans instead of new potatoes

Snacks

Vegetable sticks with guacamole or hummus

Small handful of nuts/seeds

Fresh fruit

A hard-boiled egg

Celery sticks filled with pumpkin seed butter

Olives

Exercise

A number of studies have also demonstrated that women with PCOS or insulin resistance can greatly benefit from regular exercise. For example, a study conducted at the University of Adelaide in Australia showed that a six-month programme of diet and exercise helped 18 overweight PCOS women normalise their hormones. In particular, the exercise helped to re-sensitise body cells to insulin. This helped to lower the women's overall insulin levels, helping them to lose weight and aiding in rebalancing their other hormones. In fact, the most effective kind of exercise has been found to be exercising at high intensity for at least 20 minutes, five times a week.

Support Your Metabolism

To support your diet and exercise programme, you might want to consider taking some supplements designed to support your metabolism and aid insulin sensitivity.

- A Metabolic Complex – a good metabolic complex will contain B vitamins and magnesium to support your energy levels, along with minerals, such as chromium, zinc and manganese, and herbs, such as cinnamon, fenugreek and liquorice, which help to balance blood sugar levels and re-sensitise cells to insulin.
- Alpha Lipoic Acid and Carnitine Complex – alpha lipoic acid is a powerful antioxidant that helps cells to respond better to insulin, while acetyl-l-carnitine plays an important role in fat metabolism and general heart health. For maximum support, take 2 capsules of a product supplying 200mg alpha lipoic acid and 500mg acetyl-l-carnitine, two to three times a day.
- Chromium – we've already seen in chapter 3 that the mineral chromium can be helpful for balancing blood sugar levels and improving insulin sensitivity. This makes it the perfect addition to a PCOS programme. The ideal intake for women with PCOS is 600mcg spread out through the day. It you're taking a metabolic complex as well, remember to include the chromium from this too, when working out how much extra you need.

Manage Your Heart Health

Women with PCOS often have extra fat distribution around the waist. This is significant, as this body shape (apple shape) is linked to increased incidence of many chronic health problems, including heart disease, diabetes and even asthma.

As well as a higher-than-average waist circumference, women with PCOS often also have increased blood pressure, as well as less favourable 'blood fat' profiles. Analysis of blood samples has identified that women with PCOS have higher levels of LDL or 'bad' cholesterol in their blood and lower levels of the HDL or 'good' cholesterol. This increases the risk of plaques forming in the arteries, which is a risk factor for a heart attack or stroke. The good news is that the diet and lifestyle changes mentioned above will go a long way towards helping to address these problems, but if you want to include some extra support, you could include the following:

- Fish Oil – research has shown that fish oils help to favourably alter blood fat profiles, in preference for good cholesterol. Take 2-3 1000mg capsules of high-quality omega 3 fish oil daily.

- Garlic – this is a highly popular supplement for heart health, and has been shown to lower blood pressure, as well as balancing blood cholesterol ratios. Look for a high-strength capsule containing 500mg garlic and 8000ppm allicin (the active ingredient in garlic) and take 1 capsule per day.

Become a Fan of Flax

Flax seeds are a real superfood for PCOS sufferers, as they have a number of beneficial actions. Firstly, flax seeds are a rich source of fibre and lignans. This fibre aids excess hormone elimination via the bowels, while the lignans in flax act as phytoestrogens (see chapter 15), helping to rebalance excess oestrogen levels. In addition, lignans are also able to raise the levels of sex-hormone-binding globulin, assisting the body with carrying excess hormones back to the liver for disposal.

- To get the maximum hormone-balancing effects from flax, it needs to be consumed in its cold milled form to ensure proper digestion of the fibre and lignans. Simply add one to two heaped dessertspoons to your diet each day. This can be added to smoothies, sprinkled onto fruit, salads or yoghurts or even stirred into sauces just before serving.

Balance Prolactin and Other Hormones with Agnus Castus

Agnus castus is a highly popular and effective herb used to balance many hormonal conditions, including PCOS, where the aim is to normalise progesterone levels and cycle regularity, thus suppressing the development of ovarian cysts associated with oestrogen dominance. Agnus castus is also used to help lower prolactin levels, which, as we have already noted, are often higher than normal in women with PCOS.

- For optimum support, take a supplement that provides 4mg of extract (equivalent to 28-52mg Agnus castus) daily.

Help for Excess Hair and Acne?

Research from Birmingham University (Sept 2009), has shown that both overweight and normoweight women with PCOS have higher levels of an enzyme called 5-alpha-reductase. This enzyme is used by the body to convert testosterone into its more biologically active form, DHT. It is DHT that is thought to be responsible for the acne, excessive body hair growth and also incidences of male pattern baldness that affect some women with PCOS.

What's interesting is that the action of 5-alpha-reductase is inhibited by the herb saw palmetto. This results in a reduction in levels of DHT, reducing its negative effects. But saw palmetto not only inhibits DHT production, it also inhibits it from binding to the body's hormone receptors and also helps to promote DHT degradation. This leads to reduced body hair growth and improvement in acne symptoms.

- For best results, take 1 capsule of a saw palmetto product, containing 120-160mg of extract, three times daily with meals.

Top Tip!

For further information on managing acne with diet, supplements and appropriate skin care regimes, check out the book *Nutritional Solutions for Optimising Skin Health*, available from Higher Nature (see resources page).

And Don't Forget...

As well as following the recommendations in this chapter, for a truly holistic approach, you should also read the information on liver and gut health in chapter 2 and take any steps needed to fully support these systems as well.

Chapter 6
Endometriosis

Endometriosis is more common than you might think, causing disrupted periods, pain and inflammation. But there are plenty of things that you can do to help.

Endometriosis (from endo, "inside", and metra, "womb") is a condition where cells, such as the ones in the lining of the womb, are found elsewhere in the body. According to Endometriosis UK, it affects approximately two million women in the UK (2010).

As we've seen in previous chapters, hormonal changes in the second half of a woman's reproductive cycle include a thickening of the lining of the womb. If pregnancy doesn't occur, then this lining is shed during the menstrual bleed. This is all well and good for the cells that are actually located in the womb, but when there are endometrial cells located in other places in the body, problems can occur.

Unlike a menstrual bleed, which has a clear passage out of the body, the blood released from endometriosis cells is trapped. This means that when the cells bleed each month, inflammation and pain occurs. In the long term, this can also lead to scar tissue and adhesions forming (these are where layers of body tissue, that wouldn't normally be attached, become stuck together).

Endometriosis deposits are most commonly found in locations such as on the ovary (where they form 'chocolate cysts'), inside the pelvis, in the fallopian tubes, on the outside of the womb, or on the ligaments that hold the womb in place. It can also occur on the bladder, the intestines, the vagina and the rectum and has even been found in more distant places, such as the joints and the lungs!

Symptoms of Endometriosis

The symptoms of endometriosis can vary a lot between individuals and some women have endometriosis without experiencing any symptoms at all. One of the difficulties is that in the early stages, the signs and symptoms of endometriosis appear to be the 'normal' bodily changes that take place with the menstrual cycle. It is only as time goes by that a woman begins to suspect that what is happening, and the symptoms she feels, are not normal.

The most common symptom is pelvic pain before and during periods, but there are other symptoms that can also occur:

- General, chronic pelvic pain throughout the month
- Lower back pain
- Disrupted periods – may be heavy and/or irregular
- Problems with sex/intimacy, often due to pain during intercourse
- Digestive problems, such as diarrhoea/constipation and/or painful bowel movements during menstruation
- Painful urination during menstruation
- Fatigue and lack of energy, affecting the whole body
- Headaches
- Depression, including low mood and anxiety
- Low blood sugar levels

Another symptom linked to endometriosis is infertility. This is partly because the scar tissue and adhesions that can form in endometriosis can interfere with the proper function of woman's reproductive organs. However, it has been suggested that endometriotic lesions may release factors that are detrimental to the sperm, egg or embryo.

What Causes Endometriosis?

Endometriosis is an oestrogen-dependent condition and is therefore most likely to occur during a woman's reproductive years. In fact, in experiments, oestrogen has been needed to induce or maintain endometriosis, so medical therapy is often aimed at lowering oestrogen levels to manage the condition.

In addition, there are many theories about how endometriosis can come about in the first place. Perhaps the most common explanation involves 'retrograde menstruation', which suggests that some endometrial debris, released during menstruation, passes out of the uterus, through the fallopian tubes, and into the pelvic cavity, where it invades tissue as endometriosis.

Retrograde menstruation is actually very common, but most women's immune systems can clear the debris and prevent implantation and growth of the endometrial cells. What isn't yet clear is why endometriosis develops in some women and not in others. What's more, although this theory provides a plausible rationale for the formation of endometrial deposits in the pelvic cavity, it doesn't explain how endometriosis can end up in more distant locations.

To account for this, there's another theory based on the idea that cells in the embryo, which have the potential to become endometrial later in life, get displaced as the embryo grows and develops. These migrated cells then respond to hormonal triggers, mostly in reproductive years, and develop into fully functioning endometrial cells wherever they've ended up.

In addition, some scientists are looking further and suggest that factors from the environment that mimic the effects of oestrogen could also be a triggering factor in endometriosis. These include dietary sources of hormones, such as non-organic meats, as well as hormone-mimicking substances, such as pesticides and the chemicals leached from certain kinds of plastic containers. These substances are known as xenoestrogens and are explained in more detail in chapter 15.

Lastly, there also appears to be a hereditary factor, with daughters and sisters of women with endometriosis at higher risk of developing the condition. In fact, there seems to be a specific chromosome 10q26, responsible for a 5.7:1 increased risk for developing the condition compared to the general population. In addition, it's also thought that low progesterone levels may be genetic and that this could also be a contributing factor in the hormone imbalances typical of endometriosis.

Nutritional Approaches to Endometriosis

Diet

When thinking about diet and endometriosis, the key consideration is including foods that help to balance hormones, while excluding those things that raise oestrogen levels or worsen inflammation. Most of this is covered by the dietary advice in chapter 15, but if you want to maximise your health regime, you may also like to consider the following:

Avoid gluten – nutritionists who specialise in endometriosis often find that a gluten-free diet can decrease the pain experienced by endometriosis sufferers as well as improving their fertility. This is thought to be because sensitivities to wheat or gluten can interfere with the absorption of nutrients, leading to deficiencies that exacerbate hormonal imbalances, immune dysfunction and the inflammatory response.

A Gluten-Free Diet

Gluten is a component of certain grains including wheat, spelt, kamut, rye, barley and oats. It is a sticky protein, which many people find hard to digest, and is a common cause of allergy and intolerance reactions.

Coeliac disease is a condition where gluten damages the delicate lining of the small intestine, leading to malabsorption of nutrients. In the UK, the condition affects 1 in 1,000 and tends to run in families. Gluten intolerance, on the other hand, is a more common reaction in individuals who are not coeliac. Although their reaction to gluten is less severe, the presence of gluten in the diet causes irritation to the digestive tract and can impact on nutrient absorption.

Initially, adopting a gluten-free diet can seem quite daunting. The key is to read labels carefully and experiment as much as possible with the many gluten-free wholegrains available (see resources page for some useful gluten-free cookbooks).

Gluten-Free Alternatives

- Brown Rice – this can be used as a wholegrain accompaniment to a meal, or you might want to experiment with brown rice pasta or noodles. It's also possible to buy brown rice flour (which can be used very successfully for baking) and wholegrain rice cakes, which make a great snack option
- Corn – corn pasta is available in many different forms, for example, penne, spaghetti etc. Corn cakes are a useful snack option and cornflour can be used to thicken sauces. Corn taco shells are good as an occasional treat and grilled polenta can make a good alternative to bread or pasta with a meal
- Quinoa – this is actually a seed. It can be cooked and used like rice, but is also available as flakes (good for muesli or porridge) and flour
- Buckwheat – Available as wholegrain, flour, pasta and soba noodles. Buckwheat flour is very good for making pancakes or crêpes
- Millet – this couscous-like wholegrain can be used as a meal accompaniment, or the flaked version can be cooked like porridge or added to a muesli mix
- Amaranth – this tiny seed can be cooked like a grain or popped like popcorn. It's also available ground into a flour, or as flakes to add to porridge or muesli
- Potato – A useful starchy alternative to grains. Potato flour can be used to thicken sauces.
- Chestnut – chestnut flour can be used for baking. It has a naturally sweet, nutty flavour
- Tapioca – from the cassava plant, this flour can be used to thicken sauces

- Gram or chickpea flour – these can be used to make savoury pancakes and other baked goods
- Arrowroot – this is an excellent gluten-free thickener

There is now also a wide range of ready-made gluten-free foods available including flour blends, breads, crackers, sauce, cakes, biscuits and desserts. Just be aware that many of these are high in sugar and additives, so check the packets carefully and try not to rely too heavily on pre-packaged foods.

Avoid red meat – red meat is pro-inflammatory and may contain growth hormones, including oestrogen. For this reason, it's best to avoid red meat completely and limit your intake of animal foods in general. Moderate intake of fish, especially oily fish, can be beneficial, but if you want to include other animal foods, such as eggs and chicken, make sure they're lean and organic. To keep up your protein intake, ensure you eat plenty of vegetable protein sources, such as beans, lentils, nuts, seeds, seaweeds and quinoa.

Avoid dairy products – dairy products stimulate the production of inflammatory messengers in the body, which can worsen endometriosis symptoms. What's more, dairy products (even organic ones) contain traces of hormones. The primary dairy foods that you should avoid with endometriosis include milk, yoghurt and cheese, but it's also a good idea to steer clear of butter, cream and ice cream as well. If you decide to go dairy-free, it is important to choose a healthful alternative and make sure you eat plenty of other calcium-rich foods.

Healthy Dairy Alternatives

- Rice, almond, quinoa and hazelnut milks make excellent dairy alternatives
- Mashed avocado, hummus or nut/seed butters are good alternatives to cheese and butter
- Booja Booja vegan ice cream, Coconice and Coconuka are dairy-free alternatives to ice cream, made without refined sugar and additives

A note about soya: Most of the dairy replacement soya products contain unfermented soy. This can actually exacerbate endometriosis symptoms and should be avoided in favour of the alternative above where possible.

Non-Dairy, Calcium-Rich Foods

- Pak choi
- Spinach
- Seaweed
- Chestnuts
- Sesame seeds
- Quinoa
- Salmon
- Bean sprouts (raw)
- Leafy green vegetables
- Almonds
- Walnuts and walnut butter
- Sunflower seeds
- Figs
- Sardines

Supplementary Management of Endometriosis

Conventional medical treatments for endometriosis centre on balancing levels of oestrogen (for example, with progesterone therapy) and also managing pain and inflammation. But there is also very good research on supplementary approaches.

Balancing Hormones with Herbs

When it comes to balancing hormones specific to endometriosis, we are looking at effective herbal remedies, which help to decrease oestrogen levels relative to progesterone (or to raise progesterone, to counter the oestrogen).

Agnus castus is a popular herb taken by women to rebalance the levels of oestrogen and progesterone. It works on the pituitary gland, helping to normalise the output of hormones from the ovaries. Studies have shown that extracts of agnus castus can stimulate the release of luteinising hormone (LH) and inhibit the release of follicle-stimulating hormone (FSH). This helps decrease oestrogen levels and increase progesterone production. Agnus castus may also regulate prolactin secretion, which may be of benefit to women having fertility problems.

- For optimum support, take a supplement that provides 4mg of extract (equivalent to 28-52mg of agnus castus) daily

Wild yam is another useful herb for endometriosis. It contains steroidal saponins that bind to oestrogen receptors in the body in a similar way to phytoestrogens, helping to balance progesterone and oestrogen levels. The antispasmodic and anti-inflammatory properties of wild yam can also relieve the pain associated with endometriosis and help ease the digestive complaints that sometimes accompany this condition. It is available as capsules or as a cream.

- If you want to take capsules, look out for ones that combine 150mg Mexican wild yam extract with 200mg wild yam extract per capsule
- If you'd like to use a cream, make sure the product you choose contains 20% Mexican wild yam extract along with other supporting herbs, such as dong quai, agnus castus and black cohosh

Reducing Pain and Inflammation

There are also a number of natural remedies that can help to reduce inflammation and the associated pain.

Bromelain is a protein-digesting enzyme, which can reduce the production of inflammatory messengers, as well as helping to break down blood clots. It's a very popular choice post-surgery, for traumatic injuries or wounds, as well as a helpful supplement for the inflammatory symptoms that occur when endometrial tissue breaks down during the menstrual cycle.

Pain associated with endometriosis, especially pain with inflammation, can also be effectively managed using DLPA (DL-phenylalanine). This amino acid is highly effective, enhancing the body's natural painkillers – endorphins.

In addition, many of the biochemical processes the body uses to produce inflammation are mediated by free radicals. Therefore, taking supplements that help mop up free radicals, such as the powerful antioxidant astaxanthin, can help to dampen down these responses, reducing pain.

- One option for managing endometriosis symptoms is to take a combination of 200mg bromelain, 225mg DLPA and 1mg astaxanthin, three times a day between meals

As well as bromelain, DLPA and astaxanthin, vitamin E has also been shown to be successful in reducing menstrual pain, which is a common feature of endometriosis.

- To self-supplement, take 2-3 185IU capsules of a natural vitamin E supplement daily, throughout the month

Essential fatty acids, such as the omega 3 fats EPA and DHA from fish oils, and the omega 6 fat GLA from starflower oil, can also be useful because they encourage the body to form anti-inflammatory messengers rather than inflammatory ones. This can help reduce symptoms such as pain, as well as having beneficial effects on menstrual cramps.

- For best results, take 4 capsules a day of an essential fatty acid combination supplement that provides 680mg EPA, 480mg DHA and 180mg GLA, as well as other beneficial omegas, such as palmitoleic acid (omega 7) and oleic acid (omega 9)

Other Considerations

As well as symptom management, it's also important to ensure the liver and gut are healthy to maximise oestrogen metabolism, so don't forget to read chapter 3!

Chapter 7
Fibroids

When women mention fibroids, they are almost always talking about benign tumours that originate from the smooth muscle cells of the uterus. These tumours range in size and may be solitary or multiple. They're very common and can develop at any time during a woman's reproductive years. Although the exact cause isn't known, as with many female health conditions, fibroid development is greatly influenced by hormonal imbalances.

What Affects Fibroid Development?

There are many different risk factors that can contribute to fibroid development:

- Early menarche – menstrual cycles beginning at age 10 or younger
- Use of oral contraceptive pill in early teenage years (ages 13-16)
- Use of HRT – this may prevent the shrinkage of fibroids after menopause or stimulate their growth
- History of pelvic infections
- High blood pressure – this is known to damage the smooth muscle lining of the arteries, which may cause changes in the blood vessels that lead to fibroid formation
- Being overweight – this may be related to hormonal factors, such as excess oestrogen
- High intake of animal meats, saturated fat or alcohol – these all promote oestrogen production

Research also shows that there might be some genetic and hereditary cause, as first-degree relatives have a two-and-a-half- to six-times increased risk of fibroid development.

Overall, it's widely accepted that one of the key factors in fibroid development is a hormonal imbalance. At menopause, fibroids usually begin to shrink; hence, the ovarian hormones are thought to be the main culprits.

Oestrogen and progesterone can cause division in fibrocystic 'leiomyoma' cells, resulting in fibroid growth. In addition, they can also influence the level of certain other growth factors, inflammatory chemicals and hormones (such as prolactin) that might have a part to play in fibroid development and growth. Progesterone is thought to promote the growth of fibroids by increasing the production of tumour growth factors, and decreasing the production of biochemical factors, which help deal with and break down tumours. Oestrogen, on the other hand, augments the effects of progesterone by increasing the levels of additional growth factors, which encourage cell division and unusual tissue growth.

In pre-menopausal women, fibroids show that both oestrogen receptor and progesterone receptors are over-expressed (you could, in simple terms, say overactive). In fact, the extent to which this happens is linked with the incidence and the size of fibroids. In addition to this, research shows that fibroids contain enzymes that can convert hormone precursors into oestrogen.

Types of Fibroid

As fibroids grow and develop, they can cause distortions in the surrounding tissues and organs, bleeding, tissue death, calcification and cysts. There are different types, named depending on where in the reproductive system the fibroid is growing.

- Intramural fibroids are the most common type and are found on the uterine wall. They mostly don't cause any symptoms, and begin as small nodules in the muscle layer of the uterus. Over time, as they grow, they can affect the shape of the uterus.
- Subserosal uterine fibroids develop on the outer surface of the uterus and continue to grow outwards, giving the uterus a knobbly appearance. Sometimes, these fibroids may be connected to the uterus by means of a long stalk. Over time, subserosal uterine fibroids may grow quite large, but they don't typically affect the size or shape of the uterus.
- Submucosal fibroids are partially in the cavity and partially in the wall of the uterus. They can cause heavy menstrual periods, as well as bleeding between periods and reduced fertility.
- Occasionally, fibroids are found in the muscles supporting the uterus or in the wall of the cervix.

Fibroid Symptoms

In many cases, fibroids don't cause any symptoms, but if they become very large or there's a large number of submucosal fibroids present, changes can start to occur in a woman's menstrual cycle and complications may develop. The most common symptoms associated with fibroids include:

- Abnormal bleeding from the vagina e.g. between periods
- Heavy or painful periods – this can lead to nutritional deficiencies
- Abdominal discomfort – due to constipation
- Abdominal bloating
- Pain when going to the toilet, especially around the back passage, when moving the bowels
- Disturbances in urinary habits – either needing to go more often, or not being able to go
- Pain during intercourse
- Backache
- Fertility issues – due to fibroids interfering with implantation or the function of the fallopian tubes
- Complications during pregnancy – due to bleeding or interference with the position of the foetus
- Premature labour

Nutritional Approaches to Fibroids

Where management of fibroids is concerned, there are many areas where supplements and diet can be very helpful. Whether it's rebalancing hormones or managing heavy and painful periods, there are plenty of positive steps that you can take.

An overall balancing of hormones is essential for correct management of fibroids, so it's important that you understand the basics of looking after your liver, gut, stress levels and blood sugar, which have already been covered in chapters 2 and 3. Since the excess oestrogen appears to promote the growth of fibroids, it is also very important to follow a hormone-balancing diet as shown in chapter 15.

From a supplementary point of view, the underlying hormonal imbalances and symptoms of fibroids are very similar to endometriosis. Therefore, as well as reading the advice below on managing heavy periods, it's a good idea to read the sections on 'Balancing Hormones with Herbs', and 'Reducing Pain and Inflammation' in chapter 6.

Managing Heavy Periods

Excess bleeding really can take its toll on your health, leaving you feeling run down, drained and exhausted. As well as losing blood volume, you're also losing all manner of nutrients, including the vital minerals (iron, zinc and selenium) and vitamins (B vitamins and vitamins A, C and E) needed for correct hormone balance, and for the health of every body cell.

- One quick way to remedy this is to take a high-potency multinutrient that provides good levels of all the B vitamins, at least 5000IU vitamin A, 10mg iron, 10mg zinc and 30mcg selenium, as well as all the other nutrients you normally find in a multi.

If your periods are very heavy, you might also need an extra iron supplement. This is because, over time, excess bleeding can lead to anaemia. This not only makes you feel tired, but can also cause symptoms such as pallor, irritability, breathlessness and an irregular heart beat. What's more, a lack of iron greatly impacts immune function, making you even more prone to getting run down and less likely to be able to fight off infection. Ironically, iron deficiency can also increase the risk of heavy bleeding during menstruation, because iron helps the blood vessels to contract, which is needed to slow down the flow during your periods.

- Before taking extra iron supplements, it's best to check you're genuinely deficient by arranging a blood test with your GP. If tests suggest that you need some extra iron, then it's best to take 15-20mg extra iron in a gentle, organic from that is easy to absorb, as well as including more iron-rich foods in your diet. It's also vital to decrease any food components that deplete iron uptake in the gut.

Iron-Rich Foods

- Beef
- Venison
- Seafood
- Lentils
- Pumpkin seeds
- Prunes
- Turkey
- Sardines
- Eggs
- Sesame seeds
- Dark green leafy vegetables
- Dried apricots

Iron Absorption Inhibitors

The following foods and drinks interfere with iron absorption and should be reduced or completely avoided to support optimum iron uptake:

- Red wine
- Coffee
- Tea
- Fizzy drinks
- Bran
- Unfermented soy products

Another nutrient worth increasing, whether you're iron deficient or not, is vitamin C. That's because vitamin C is essential for the body to absorb iron from food or supplements, as well as being a key nutrient for strengthening blood vessels to reduce excess bleeding.

To benefit from these effects, take 1000mg vitamin C with 500mg bioflavonoids daily. If you're taking iron supplements, you should take the two together on an empty stomach for optimum absorption.

Chapter 8
Thrush

It's a strange name for a fungal infection, thrush. Candidiasis sounds a little more lady-like. But whatever it's named, the symptoms of thrush can be irritating and unpleasant.

What is Thrush?

Candidiasis, or thrush, is a fungal infection caused by any of the *Candida* yeast species, of which *Candida albicans* is the most common. It's also sometimes called a yeast infection. It occurs when there is an imbalance in the natural microflora of the body, for example, in the mouth, the vagina or the gastrointestinal tract. It can affect everyone from young babies through to people in older age, but vaginal candidiasis is particularly common in women of reproductive years.

Symptoms and Causes of Thrush

Candida thrives on moist surfaces, which explains why it's found in such body areas as the mouth and vagina. These are excellent environments for it to grow and breed, but usually, the number of *Candida* is kept in check by the immune system and friendly bacteria. The problem is, *Candida* is an opportunistic pathogen. This means that under the right conditions, such as a compromised immune system or change in friendly bacteria levels, *Candida* can quickly overgrow, causing the symptoms of an infection.

What's more, hormonal disturbances can affect a woman's chance of developing candidiasis. For example, it has been noted that women who are pregnant, on oral contraceptives or on hormone replacement therapy might be more prone to thrush compared to other women. Diabetics and those who have had a long course of antibiotics are also at increased risk.

Typical symptoms include:

- Itching of affected area
- Soreness and redness (local inflammation)
- Discomfort in the vagina
- Severe burning sensation with whitish-grey discharge

Conventional Management of Thrush

While conventional treatments for thrush nearly always involve anti-yeast medications, such as fluconazole, which aim to get rid of the yeast in one fell swoop, nutritional and natural health alternatives take a little longer. This is because holistic practices believe in not just treating the symptoms, but also the cause. For this reason, naturopathic approaches to thrush will not only look at agents which have been proven to effectively clear the yeast infection, but also look at immune system health and dietary measures which might affect the growth of *Candida*.

Supplementary Management of Thrush

For women who have had multiple treatments with anti-yeast medication, or who might have reacted to them, natural alternatives are often very welcome. Some women choose to try natural alternatives first, and to maintain the regime long-term to safeguard against reoccurrence if they are prone to this condition.

Natural Antimicrobials

Garlic

Well-known for its antimicrobial properties, clinical studies have shown that garlic can inhibit the growth of *Candida*. Do remember though, that research is most often carried out based on supplements, so while adding fresh garlic into your diet is useful, you would need a lot of it to get a clinical effect.

- To get the full benefits from garlic, look for a 500mg garlic supplement providing 8000ppm allicin, 20000ppm alliin and 8500ppm thiosulfinates. Take 1 capsule a day until your symptoms have been clear for five days

Octanoic acid

Octanoic acid, or caprylic acid as it is often known, is a natural anti-fungal agent which helps to kill *Candida* and maintain a healthy balance of friendly bacteria in the body.

- Two capsules of a good supplement will include 350mg calcium octanoate and 350mg magnesium octanoate, along with the supportive action of herbs such as pau d'arco, thyme, rosemary and lemon balm. Take 1 capsule with each main meal

Probiotics

Probiotics are often recommended for cases of thrush, because changes in the body's balance of friendly bacteria in the gut or vagina can cause the internal environment to become more favourable for *Candida*, allowing it to overgrow. Because of this, it makes sense to include friendly bacteria that will compete for space and food, and by default, oust unwanted bacteria and yeasts.

Since candidiasis may be present in the gut at the same time as in the vagina, it's best to combine oral probiotic supplements with vaginal probiotics. It is especially important to take a course of probiotics after having antibiotics, as these will have wiped out the good bacteria that should be present in your gut.

- For oral supplementation, take a high-potency supplement providing a daily dose of 9 billion of the most researched probiotic strains for at least one month
- To restore microflora balance in the vagina, some women find a pessary containing friendly bacteria from the *Lactobacilli* family helpful. Look for a pessary containing 5 billion organisms (preferably a mix of *L. acidophilus, L. plantarum, L. rhamnosus, casei* and *L. bulgaricus*) and insert 1 capsule each night for 10 nights

Echinacea

If your immune system is compromised, you might want to consider the herbal remedy echinacea. This is sometimes recommended to women with thrush, as it helps the body's white blood cells to manage infection more efficiently.

- A good therapeutic dose is 176mg echinacea dried juice (20-28:1) (equivalent to up to 4928mg echinacea) twice per day until the infection has been cleared for five days

What About Diet?

Low sugar?

While conventional *Candida* treatments give you a large hit of anti-yeast medication, they ask nothing in the way of a diet change, so once their effects have worn off, you may still be encouraging yeast overgrowth because of what you are eating. You are left with the same poor dietary habits, all of which could have encouraged *Candida* in the first place.

Instead, it's important to think holistically, and try to reduce the sugar in your diet, as this is the main food source for the *Candida*. This means avoiding sugar itself, as well as all foods containing sugar, such as biscuits, cakes, pastries and confectionery, as well as fizzy drinks and alcohol. It would also be wise to look at your intake of white, refined carbohydrates, such as bread, rice and pasta, as these quickly break down into sugar in the digestive tract and will promote thrush.

- Cutting out all visual sugar and following the hormone-balancing diet in chapter 15 is an excellent place to start

Mushrooms and Yeast?

In principle, you can eat food yeasts and mushrooms, as they don't colonise your gut like *Candida* and its relatives. However, some people with *Candida* experience a cross-reaction against mushrooms and foods containing yeast. In these cases, it's best to avoid these foods until your infection has cleared up. As well as baked goods, such as bread, yeast is also found in some stock cubes and in foods such as Marmite. If you are not sure whether you are sensitive to yeast and mushrooms, it's probably best to reduce or avoid these foods as a precaution.

Chapter 9
Cystitis

When you think of 'cystitis', you might associate this with a urinary tract infection, and you'd be right. But there are other kinds of cystitis that you should also be aware of.

What is Cystitis?

Cystitis is the name given to urinary bladder inflammation, and in layperson's terms, most often describes a urinary tract infection. But this isn't the only cause. Sometimes, damage to the tissues of the bladder, and its various networks of tubes, can result in bladder inflammation, too. In fact, this is far more common than urinary tract infections.

Traumatic cystitis, the most common form of cystitis in women, is due to 'bruising' of the bladder, usually from sexual intercourse. This is often followed by bacterial cystitis, as bacteria from the bowel find their way through the urethra into the bladder. In sexually active women, the most common culprits are the bacteria *E. coli* and *Staphylococcus saprophyticus*.

Interstitial cystitis is another type of cystitis, which, in this instance, is a result of an actual injury to the bladder, which causes constant irritation. It rarely involves a bacterial infection. As the symptoms are similar to a urinary tract infection, often, conventional treatments are given, only for symptoms to persist after urinary analysis confirms a normal bacterial count. As a result, antibiotics might have been inappropriately prescribed. Exactly why some women are prone to interstitial cystitis is unknown, though some scientists point to an autoimmune link.

Symptoms of cystitis:

- Painful urination
- Frequent urination
- Urgent need to urinate
- Abnormal urine colour – cloudy – similar to urinary tract infection
- Blood in the urine
- Strong-smelling, or foul-smelling urine
- Feeling of pressure in the lower pelvis

Natural Management of Cystitis

Cystitis is one example of a well-researched health condition where even conventional practitioners actively encourage natural remedies. One reason for this is that it has captured the attention of large food producers, who are keen to fund research to show that their cranberry juice, for example, can positively impact on cystitis. These studies have shown that components in cranberry can help prevent the *E. coli* bacteria from sticking to the wall of the urinary tract, thus preventing a urinary tract infection.

Use Cranberry Appropriately

The problem with many of the cranberry-containing drinks is that they contain a great deal of sugar, which has a detrimental effect on the immune system. A good alternative is either to source an unsweetened cranberry juice or use a cranberry extract supplement. This includes cranberry in a high concentration, and is most appropriate for anyone with an actual urinary tract infection.

- Look for a supplement containing at least 500mg whole concentrated cranberry and take 2 capsules a day

Change Urinary pH

Although many practitioners believe that acidifying the urine is the best approach to addressing cystitis, alkalising the urine has in fact been shown to be more effective, especially in women with an active bacterial infection. The best way to achieve this is to supplement with alkalising mineral salts. A good blend will contain a mixture of magnesium carbonate, sodium bicarbonate and potassium bicarbonate, and pH strips are often provided so you can monitor the alkalising effects on your urine.

- If using a powder, stir one heaped teaspoon into a glass of water and drink between meals

- If using capsules, take five on an empty stomach with a glass of water

Helpful Herbals

Oregano

The oil from the herb oregano is one of nature's most powerful antiseptics. It contains the active ingredient carvacrol, which is a natural antimicrobial agent, capable of killing a wide range of bacteria, yeasts, fungi and other microorganisms. In particular, carvacrol has potent antibacterial activity against *E. coli*, one of the most common causes of UTIs. As an added bonus, oregano oil also has beneficial anti-inflammatory and immune-system-supporting effects as well.

- To harness these effects, take a supplement containing 50mg pure oregano oil three times a day with meals

Echinacea

If you are constantly experiencing urinary tract infections, it makes sense to review your immune status. Though echinacea's immune-enhancing ability does not directly involve an anti-microbial action itself, it will help your body to better manage an infection.

- A good dose is 176mg echinacea dried juice (20-28:1) (equivalent to up to 4928mg echinacea) twice per day

Dealing with Soreness and Inflammation

Whether cystitis has been caused by a UTI or some kind of irritation or injury to the bladder, remedies that help to reduce soreness and inflammation are always welcome!

- Vitamin E is one of the most popular supplements for soreness and, taken at 400iu daily long-term, can be highly effective
- As well as this, take a daily dose of a high-potency antioxidant formulation, including vitamins C and A and minerals zinc and selenium, to counter the effects of inflammation
- Essential fatty acids are also a must for anyone wanting to manage inflammatory reactions, especially the omega 3 essential fats, which are most commonly found in fish and flax seed oils. Opt for 3000mg of a high-quality fish oil or two tablespoons of cold pressed organic flax oil each day

Chapter 10
Menstrual Irregularities

While most women's menstrual cycles follow a pattern of anything from 21 to 35 days, many factors can alter the length of time in between a woman's period and some women don't menstruate at all. For those that do, periods can range anywhere from a painless, light blood flow to a heavy or painful ordeal. This chapter looks at why these irregularities might occur and what could help.

Irregular Periods

While some women find that their menstrual cycles are regular, others simply don't know when the next one is going to arrive. Not only does this make the necessary preparations impossible (when are you going to feel tired, or irritable, for example?), it can also influence conception, as ovulation is so much harder to predict. Any variation in cycle length that is plus or minus four days is said to be medically 'normal'. However, any variation of between eight and 20 days is considered moderately irregular, and more than this is considered very irregular.

An irregular length of time between periods is termed metrorrhagia. Cycle lengths of shorter than 21 days, or longer than 36 days, are considered irregular. Infrequent or very light menstruation is termed oligomenorrhoea. Irregular periods are diagnosed when this has occurred for several months and they can be caused by many factors: stress; thyroid and liver problems; changes in eating patterns and excessive exercising; hormone-related conditions, such as PCOS, endometriosis, fibroids and cysts; and onset of the menopause.

Heavy Periods

The term menorrhagia is used to describe abnormally heavy and prolonged periods. From month to month, women get to know their 'normal' (or, as we should say, 'typical') amount of menstrual bleed. On average, women lose 25-80ml of blood over a period of five days (as a guide, a regular tampon usually holds about 5ml of blood). A blood loss of over 80ml, or a menstrual flow lasting over seven days, constitutes menorrhagia. This may occur in a regular or irregular pattern.

Many different factors can cause periods to become heavier, and often, with this, more painful. Excessive build-up of the endometrial lining can be a causal factor, which is common in conditions where ovulation might become delayed, or eggs aren't fully developed. When this occurs, less progesterone is produced and oestrogen can freely keep building up the uterine lining. Thus, it stands to reason that any condition where there is an imbalance in normal ratios of progesterone to oestrogen can result in heavy bleeding. This situation can also occur just before the menopause and explains why some perimenopausal women experience unusually heavy menstrual flow in the last few cycles before their periods stop.

Fibroids in the wall of the womb can also cause increased menstrual loss, especially if they protrude into the central cavity, increasing the surface area of the endometrium, while extensions into the womb wall caused by endometriosis may increase blood loss and pain on menstruation.

Painful Periods

Painful periods, or dysmenorrhoea, affects more than 50% of menstruating females, with around 10-12% of them experiencing pain so bad that it disrupts their lives for one to three days each month. Dysmenorrhoea is very common in young women between the ages of 20 and 24, though it can affect women at any age (it is a myth that having children eases period pain). Risk factors include starting your periods early, having long periods, being overweight and smoking.

Period pain is often categorised as either primary or secondary dysmenorrhoea:

Primary dysmenorrhoea usually begins a few hours before or just after the onset of menstruation, with the cramps most severe on day one and/or two of bleeding. These typically affect the lower abdomen, the back and the inner thighs (like labour pain) and usually last for two to three days. Research has shown that women who experience period pain tend to produce abnormal levels of inflammatory messengers called prostaglandins (eight to 13 times that of women who don't experience period pain). This results in abnormal amounts of pain, increased number of uterine contractions and dysrhythmic uterine activity, especially in the first 48 hours of the period.

Secondary dysmenorrhoea is period pain as a result of an underlying condition, such as endometriosis, pelvic inflammatory disease, polyps and adhesions, ovarian cysts, and malformations of the womb or cervix (often accompanied by a tendency not to ovulate). Research has also shown that women with an IUD may have localised reactions that result in an increase in prostaglandin release (and sometimes an increase in bleeding too), similar to primary dysmenorrhoea.

Contributing Factors

Stress

Stress can greatly influence hormonal balance because when we're under stress, our bodies release increased levels of the hormone cortisol. The downside of this is that cortisol can reduce the effects of luteinising hormone, oestradiol (the active form of oestrogen) and progesterone. What's more, when the biochemical pathways to switch cortisol production on are activated, it can suppress the signals needed to stimulate ovulation, stopping this from occurring. Aside from general stress, patients with clinical depression may also have raised cortisol levels as well.

Thyroid Imbalances

Thyroid problems can cause menstrual cycle irregularity, with oligomenorrhoea and amenorrhoea (a lack of periods) commonly occurring in patients with an overactive thyroid (hyperthyroidism), while an underactive thyroid (hypothyroidism) is associated with an irregular cycle and heavier periods. With hyperthyroidism, there is an increase in the level of sex-hormone-binding globulin, which can disturb the delicate balance of circulating hormones. With hypothyroidism, problems are mainly as a result of increased prolactin levels. This increase in prolactin happens 'accidently' when the pituitary gland is trying to stimulate the thyroid.

Liver Health

From previous chapters, we have read how compromised liver function can lead to hormonal disruption. In fact, alcohol has a profound effect on female reproduction. Research from the United States has shown that female alcoholics aged 20-40 have a decreased number of ovarian follicles and no corpus lutea, causing menstrual irregularities and even lack of ovulation.

Significant Changes in Weight and Exercise

Maintaining a healthy, stable weight is vital, because both severe weight loss or weight gain can result in menstrual irregularities, including the inability to ovulate. Severe weight loss leads to a reduction in the level of active oestrogen, leading to a thinning of the endometrial lining in the womb. In addition, reduced body fat levels correspond with a lower output of the hormone leptin, which can lead to a lack of ovulation.

Research has shown that 50% of bulimics have amenorrhoea and that this is associated with decreased levels of luteinising hormone, which occur when body weight drops by 15% or more. In fact, amenorrhea can occur in any woman who loses 10-15% of their normal body weight. This is especially true if the weight loss is accompanied by aggressive exercise, as this raises cortisol levels, which can interfere with ovulation.

But it's not just underweight women who don't ovulate. Fat tissue produces both androgens and oestrogen, so obesity can result in excess testosterone and oestrogen in the body and reduced progesterone. There are other changes in hormones with obesity too, such as decreased levels of follicle-stimulating hormone and prolactin. This influences a woman's ability to ovulate and, therefore, her menstrual regularity. The good news is that these negative hormonal changes are reversed when weight is lost.

Onset of Menopause

As women approach the menopause, their hormone balance changes, which can result in irregular periods, as well as unpredictable amounts of menstrual bleed. This is due to decreasing production of oestrogen and progesterone. As levels of oestrogen become inconsistent, the thickness of the endometrium can change, leading to unpredictable and heavy bleeding. Progesterone's role, on the other hand, is to trigger the shedding of the uterine contents after ovulation, so as progesterone levels decline, irregular periods can result. It's also common for women reaching menopause to ovulate more erratically, often not ovulating at all. This results in a pronounced decrease in progesterone, which can then cause an oestrogen surge and further menstrual irregularities.

Menstrual Irregularities – A Holistic Approach

Conventional treatments for menstrual irregularities often involve using the oral contraceptive pill to maintain an artificial but regular bleed and anti-inflammatories to manage the pain. But frequently, women prefer to try more natural approaches to manage their symptoms.

Helpful Herbs

Agnus castus

Studies on agnus castus have shown good results in women suffering with irregular and/or heavy periods. It works on the pituitary gland, helping to regulate ovulation and, therefore, progesterone levels. In one study, 126 women were supplemented with agnus castus on a long-term basis. In the 33 women with a short menstrual cycle, supplementation increased the average cycle length from 20 to 26 days, while the same treatment in a group of 35 women with a longer-than-normal menstrual cycle caused their average cycle to shorten from 39 to 31 days. For the 58 women with heavy periods, Agnus castus supplementation decreased the duration of bleeding from eight to five days.

- For best effects, take a supplement that provides 4mg of extract (equivalent to 28-52mg of agnus castus) daily on an ongoing basis. Since hormones run on a monthly cycle, it can take six months or more for your cycle to reset

Ginger

Ginger has powerful circulation-increasing properties and is also a potent anti-inflammatory. This is one reason why it is so popular for painful periods. Home remedies have been traditionally taken, but a supplement is preferable to ensure you get a significant dose.

In 2009, scientists carried out a study to investigate the menstrual pain-relieving effects of ginger tablets compared to ibuprofen and mefenamic acid. They asked a group of 150 female students who regularly suffered with menstrual pain to take either four 250mg doses of ginger tablets, 250mg mefenamic acid or 400mg ibuprofen. The tablets were taken for the first three days of the menstrual period and the women were asked to rate the severity of their symptoms. When the results were analysed, the scientists found that the ginger tablets were as effective as the conventional pain relief medication!

- If you want to use this natural alternative, take 300mg ginger standardised extract (5% gingerols) three to four times a day on the days you normally experience period pain

Managing Muscle Cramping

To help manage menstrual cramps, magnesium is a most amazing mineral. Research has shown that it can act on many types of muscle, especially smooth muscles such as those found in the uterus. It is actively needed for muscle relaxation and studies have shown that it can help reduce painful period cramps.

- A good dose to take is the equivalent of 200mg of an easy-to-absorb form of magnesium, three times daily

Whole-Body Support

For more information on calming down pain and inflammation, follow the suggestions in chapter 6 on endometriosis. If you suffer with heavy periods, you should also check out chapter 7 on fibroids, which contains important information on the nutrients you need to help your body rebuild its blood stores.

As well as these specific steps, please also read chapters 2 and 3, to see the importance of maintaining a healthy liver and digestive tract, as well as a healthy blood sugar balance, and aiding stress reduction.

Chapter 11
Fibrocystic Breast Disease

Fibrocystic breast disease, as the name suggests, is a condition where non-cancerous lumps appear in the breasts, causing pain and discomfort (an older name for the condition is chronic cystic mastitis, which gives you some idea of the discomfort which can result).

Various research papers suggest that fibrocystic breast disease affects between 30% and 60% of women at various times in their life. It is a common condition and is often influenced by hormonal changes during the menstrual cycle, so some have questioned whether 'disease' is really the right terminology for it.

Fibrocystic breast disease involves the glandular breast tissue. The sole known biologic function of these glands is the production and secretion of milk. They occupy a major portion of the breast and are surrounded by fatty tissue and other support elements. The glandular tissue itself is composed of different types of cells, including clusters of secretory cells that produce milk, and cells that line the surfaces of the secretory cells, called the epithelial cells.

In fibrocystic breast disease, there are abnormal changes in the breast tissue, including the development of fibrous lumps and a 'cobblestone'-like appearance and texture. The lumps are smooth with clearly defined edges and can most often move around. These can appear near the surface, or deeper down in the breast tissue (making them harder to detect), but the most common site is in the upper and outer area of the breast near to the armpit. Often, the first symptoms include an ache in the breasts, with swelling and tenderness (sometimes with itching) and nipple symptoms, such as increased sensitivity. Of course, these are often premenstrual symptoms too, which in part explains why there is a link to hormonal changes at various points in the menstrual cycle, especially just before a woman's period.

The most common culprits in fibrocystic breast disease are the hormones oestrogen and progesterone (though other hormones, such as prolactin, insulin and thyroid hormones, can all affect the breast tissue, too). As well as preparing the uterus for a pregnancy, these hormones also prepare the breast tissue for lactation each month by stimulating cell growth and increasing the activity of blood vessels, cell metabolism and the supporting tissues. All this activity may contribute to the feeling of breast fullness and fluid retention that women commonly experience before their menstrual period.

However, when the monthly cycle is over, these stimulated breast cells cannot simply slough away like the uterus lining. Instead, the breast cells have to undergo a process of programmed cell death, called apoptosis. During this process, enzymes are activated that break down the breast cells from within. The resulting cellular fragments are then further broken down by inflammatory cells and nearby glandular cells. During this process, the fragments of broken cells and the inflammation caused by the clean-up operation may lead to scarring (fibrosis) that damages the tissues within the breast. Over many years, this can result in the breast tissue becoming dense or fibrous. This typically occurs after the age of 30 (and often after pregnancy), resulting in an increase in breast pain and the development of small cysts. Generally speaking, larger cysts don't usually appear until after age 35 or so, and by the time a woman reaches the menopause, symptoms usually subside, as her levels of oestrogenic hormones diminish.

Rather than being a simple condition, with a prescribed set of symptoms, fibrocystic breast disease is often complicated. The degree to which hormones affect the breast, and even different areas of the breast, can vary, as can the degree of inflammation, and the extent to which cyclical hormones affect symptoms. For many, a truly holistic, complete-body approach is the best way to manage the condition, which improves overall health, too.

Symptoms of Fibrocystic Breast Disease:

- Tenderness in a breast/the breasts
- Prolonged discomfort in a breast/the breasts
- Dull pain
- Lumpy breasts/nodular breasts

A Bit About Breast Cancer

The symptoms associated with fibrocystic breast disease can sometimes cause concern because they are very similar to the first signs of breast cancer. For this reason, any changes in breast tissue should always be checked over by a GP.

However, it is worthwhile noting that the risk of a more serious complication is actually very low. In fact, only 5% of women with fibrocystic breast disease have the type of cellular changes that can develop into breast cancer. While women with this condition might be told that their risk of developing breast cancer is higher than other woman in the population (an increased risk of two to six per cent over their lifetime), the actual risk of developing breast cancer in any given year is still comparatively low.

Natural Approaches for Fibrocystic Breast Disease

The symptoms of painful, tender breasts (usually in the week leading up to menstruation) is most often linked with a higher ratio of oestrogen compared to progesterone (if women are experiencing irregular periods, then it's likely that an under-production of progesterone is present). Some women have normal amounts of progesterone, but their tissue might be more sensitive to oestrogen or a hormonal imbalance may be causing fluid retention in the breast.

Balancing Hormones with Phytoestrogens

As well as following the dietary advice in chapter 15, there are many supplements that you can choose to help balance hormones, but with fibrocystic breast disease, balancing oestrogen levels is the most important factor.

It is interesting to note that Asian women tend not to suffer with hormonal problems, such as breast discomfort and, indeed, their incidence of breast cancer is very low. This is thought to be because their traditional diets are very high in plant oestrogens. Found in foods such as fermented soya products, chickpeas and lentils, these natural phytoestrogens are weakly oestrogenic and have an oestrogen-balancing effect in the body. They bind to oestrogen receptors in tissues, including breast tissue, thus blocking out powerfully active body oestrogen. The overall result is a dampening down of oestrogen activity in the body, and an improvement of symptoms over time.

- Taking a daily supplement containing 1000mg of high-potency, fermentation-activated whole soya, providing a total of 40mg isoflavones per tablet, is recommended

Manage Pain with Vitamin E and Starflower Oil

Vitamin E is a highly popular supplement for all manner of breast pain and discomfort, and has been for many, many years. Initial observations that vitamin E is useful for breast disease were explained in the 1960s, where women with cyclical and non-cyclical breast symptoms reported positive results for tenderness and pain.

- You need around 400-800iu of vitamin E daily, for a period of at least two months, to get the full benefits

Another popular choice is starflower oil, which is a rich source of the essential fatty acid, gamma-linolenic acid (GLA). It contains almost three times as much of this beneficial nutrient than evening primrose oil! GLA is of interest in fibrocystic breast disease because research has shown that it can reduce the symptoms of breast tenderness, including inflammation and swelling. This is because in the body, GLA is converted into hormone-like prostaglandins, which regulate a number of bodily functions, including hormonal balance and inflammation.

- For the first three months, take two 1000mg capsules of starflower oil containing at least 200mg GLA daily. After this, a maintenance dose of one capsule a day is recommended

Avoid Methylxanthines

Coffee, chocolate, tea, soft drinks, wine, beer and some over-the-counter medications contain caffeine or other similar compounds (collectively called methylxanthines) that can trigger the body to increase production of stress hormones. This can cause fluid retention in the breast and exacerbate breast lumps and tenderness. Studies have shown that reducing or eliminating these foods from the diet can diminish symptoms in up to 80% of women.

- If you suffer with fibrocystic breast disease, it's a good idea to monitor whether these foods and drinks play a role in worsening your symptoms, by removing them for a test period of around three months

Reduce Salt

Salt increases our tendency to retain water and can contribute to breasts becoming heavy and swollen premenstrually. To combat this, it's a good idea to cut back on your salt intake two weeks before your period. This includes the salt hidden in processed foods, as well as added salt at the table or during cooking.

Eat Plenty of Natural Diuretics

Another way to help reduce the symptoms of fibrocystic breast disease is to eat foods that have a natural diuretic effect. These will help to reduce fluid retention, reducing the discomfort caused by the breast tissue swelling.

- Good choices include: celery, tomatoes, asparagus, artichokes, horseradish, parsley, apple cider vinegar, watermelon, cranberries, oats and green tea

Good Liver Health

As well as tackling specific symptoms head on, a natural health approach to fibrocystic breast disease also requires us to look at the health of the liver. After all, the liver is the primary site for oestrogen clearance and oestrogen metabolism. Thus, it stands to reason that compromised liver function can affect overall hormonal balance, and can result in changes to the breasts. Nutritional supplements can be used to improve liver function and thereby support a more balanced oestrogen metabolism. To find out more, read chapter 2.

A Healthy Digestive System

Healthy digestion is also pivotal, as hormone balance is, in part, managed in the gastro-intestinal tract. Women having fewer than three bowel movements per week have a four- to five-times increased risk of fibrocystic breast disease, compared to women having one or more bowel movements per day.

As mentioned in chapter 2, gut transit time is an important consideration, as a slow gut transit increases toxic build-up and allows excreted oestrogens to be reabsorbed. To find out more about how probiotics and colon-cleansing supplements can help, see chapter 2.

Chapter 12
Low Libido

Intimacy and sexual health are an important part of any woman's life and because it most often involves another partner, it can be the cause of many a heated 'discussion', leaving the woman in need of some sound advice.

The Biochemistry of Sexual Desire

Our response to intimacy and sexual signals are an inherent part of our being human. It's biochemical to the core, and also involves many aspects of the way we think and feel. Sexual desire and arousal are a sequence of very finely tuned hormonal and neurological events, so it stands to reason that these patterns can sometimes get out of 'sync'.

While we can excuse a lack of lust and a rushing pulse at the sight of our partners when they walk in the door (a little familiar), what is happening when a lack of sexual interest lasts for weeks, and the weeks become months? It helps to look a little deeper.

Hot-blooded testosterone. It's the hormone of lust, which drives men towards sexual prowess; the 'I want it now' response that powers sexual acts. But, for women, testosterone alone is not enough. It's the combination of oestrogen and testosterone together that is important for female desire.

In the female body, testosterone is naturally produced in small amounts by the ovaries and typically surges a few days before ovulation. This increase in testosterone, along with rising levels of oestrogen, causes sexual desire to peak – a driver for female interest in males to encourage copulation. This change in hormones also increases the release of libido-enhancing neurotransmitters in the brain, such as dopamine and serotonin.

There have been many studies on the biochemistry of sexual desire and arousal, charting when, and at which point of, the 'first look' turns into 'first lust', and then arousal, and ultimately (though not, some argue, so importantly), orgasm. Researchers have shown that women respond well to visual stimuli, but that this doesn't necessarily lead to the need for intercourse.

While desire is complicated, arousal is relatively straightforward. As with men, once the desire is there, women's bodies follow suit with physiological responses. There is increased vaginal blood flow, lubrication of the vaginal tract, enlargement of the breasts, increase in the size of the nipples, dilation of the pupils, an increase in heart rate and flushing of the skin.

After the menopause, when oestrogen levels naturally decrease, these responses can alter. Symptoms such as hot flushes and vaginal dryness, fatigue and changes in mood can all affect libido, and sexual desire can diminish. But this doesn't have to be the case! These symptoms can be overcome, often by rebalancing hormone levels in the body or using vaginal lubricants so that sexual life can once again become fulfilling.

When Things Go Wrong...

Sexual desire can be affected by mental and emotional factors, as well as physical changes, illness and medications. Common issues include:

- Painful sex (dyspareunia)
- Inability to orgasm (anorgasmia)
- Inhibitions
- Cultural or religious attitudes towards sex
- Adverse effects of medications – these include medications such as those used to treat the heart, arthritis, cancer, diabetes or neurological conditions, as well as antihistamines and antidepressants, both of which have been shown to reduce sexual desire
- Body changes related to breasts or genital areas can affect perceptions of body image, and desire for sex – whether 'natural' or due to surgeries
- Alcohol/drugs – may depress sexual drive over time
- Fatigue – lack of sleep physiologically affects desire, on a biochemical as well as perceived level
- Hormonal changes – e.g. during the menopause, or during/after pregnancy
- Stress – stress hormones can interfere with hormonal balance, which can lead to a reduction in libido (as well as tiredness and lack of 'feel good' chemicals, such as dopamine and serotonin, which encourage desire)
- Poor circulation or blood flow to the sexual organs
- Issues with a partner – lack of connection, unresolved conflicts, infidelity, poor communication of sexual needs and preferences

Natural Solutions to Increase Libido

Conventional approaches to low libido in women often concentrate on supplementing oestrogen levels to positively increase desire and mood. That's because although testosterone is an important driver in desire, testosterone replacement therapies can lead to women developing male characteristics, such as excess hair (hirsutism) or acne. Natural medicine, on the other hand, takes a more holistic approach to boosting libido, aiming to balance hormones, reduce stress and boost circulation.

Boost Desire with Damiana

Damiana is a South American herb, well known for its libido-enhancing qualities and positive effects on the reproductive organs. The herb reduces stress and anxiety and produces a feeling of relaxation and mild euphoria. It also helps to balance female hormone levels.

- A good dose is 450mg of damiana aphrodisiaca standardised extract, twice a day away from meals

Balance Your Mood

Look out for supplements that can help to naturally encourage production of neurotransmitters, such as dopamine, which are important for feelings of desire. The amino acid tyrosine is particularly useful as it not only aids the production of dopamine, but also noradrenalin, which is associated with alertness, happiness and motivation – all vital for sexual desire.

- To get the full effects, you need a supplement containing at least 500mg tyrosine, along with all the cofactor nutrients required for neurotransmitter production. These include vitamins C, B6 and B12, niacin and folic acid, as well as the minerals zinc and manganese

Encourage Healthy Blood Flow

As we've seen above, blood flow is an important part of female arousal. The problem is that poor circulation or other factors that interfere with blood flow, such as diabetes and certain medication, can affect libido.

In the body, the process used to aid blood to flow into a particular area is a widening of the blood vessels. This is triggered by the release of a substance called nitric oxide, which relaxes the blood vessel walls so more blood can flow through them. The problem is that when the blood vessels have been damaged by high blood pressure, high sugar levels, excess cholesterol or smoking, the ability to make nitric oxide decreases.

One way to counter this is to take a supplement containing the amino acid arginine. Often touted as a natural alternative to Viagra, arginine supports the production of nitric oxide in the body, improving blood flow to the sexual organs. For women, L-arginine can enhance the arousal process and may even improve orgasm.

- For best results, take 3000mg arginine in combination with phosphatidyl choline and pantothenic acid, 30 minutes before sex. The phosphatidyl choline and pantothenic acid enhance the production of acetylcholine, which is a neurotransmitter important for sexual response

Exercise

Exercise is well known to increase levels of feel-good neurotransmitters in the brain and boost circulation, so it makes sense to include some purposeful physical exercise each week (5 x 30 minutes is recommended). This will not only help you to feel better, but it will also help keep you supple and strong in the bedroom. Add into this some pelvic floor exercises, and you will know that you're ready for action, when it arises.

Avoid Alcohol

While one alcoholic drink could help you to relax and lose your inhibitions, too much compromises emotion, mood and bedroom performance. What's more, in the long term, alcohol can affect the function of the liver, making it less effective at clearing oestrogen, which can lead to the significant hormonal imbalance that lowered libido in the first place.

Chapter 13
Hair Loss

While it is generally accepted that men lose their hair as they age, hair loss can also affect women, occurring at a variety of different life stages.

Different Types of Hair Loss

Telogen Effluvium

This is one of the commonest forms of hair loss in women and refers to a condition where there is diffuse (or widely spread out) shedding of the hair from both the scalp and elsewhere on the body. This can occur at any age and generally starts quite suddenly, although most cases resolve themselves within six months.

Normal hair growth cycles alternate between a three-year growth phase, called anagen, and a three-month resting phase, called telogen. At any one time, up to about 15% of hairs are in telogen. During this time, the hair usually remains in the follicle until they're pushed out by the growth of a new hair.

In telogen effluvium, a sudden stress on the body, hormone imbalance or sometimes a reaction to a medication, can trigger large numbers of hairs to enter the telogen phase at the same time. This results in widespread shedding about three months later. Once the new hairs start to grow again, the density of hair often improves and starts to thicken again.

Androgenetic Alopecia

Another common type of hair loss in women is androgenetic alopecia. This affects roughly 50% of men (where it causes male pattern baldness) and perhaps as many women over the age of 40. It is caused by a hormone imbalance, but the tendency to develop the condition has a genetic basis, often being inherited from the father or mother.

The cause of hair loss in androgenetic alopecia is a chemical called dihydrotestosterone, or DHT. This can be produced in the body from testosterone by the action of an enzyme called 5-alpha reductase. People with a lot of this enzyme make more DHT, which in excess, can cause the hair follicles to make thinner and thinner hair, until eventually, they stop working completely.

In women, the pattern of hair loss is different to the typical receding hairline and central balding in men. Instead, androgenetic alopecia causes a general thinning of women's hair, with loss predominantly over the top and sides of the head. This hair loss makes the scalp more visible and, if you have a parting, this will often look wider.

Alopecia Areata

Another important cause of hair loss in women is a condition called alopecia areata. This is an autoimmune disease, where the hair follicles are attacked by the immune system. This causes the follicles to become very small, slowing hair production to the point that there may be no visible hair growth for months, or years.

After some time, hair may regrow as before, come back in patchy areas, or not regrow at all. The good news is that in every case, the hair follicles remain alive and can be switched on again; the bad news is that we don't yet know how to do this.

Contributing Factors

PCOS – women who have PCOS tend to have higher levels of DHT than women who are unaffected. This can lead to androgenetic alopecia that typically occurs in a woman's mid- to late-20s. For more information on this condition, see chapter 5.

Pregnancy – many women notice hair loss about three months after they've had a baby. This is because the high levels of certain hormones produced during pregnancy cause the body to keep hair that would normally fall out. When the hormones return to pre-pregnancy levels, that hair falls out, but then the normal cycle of growth and loss starts again so this kind of hair loss doesn't require any further treatment.

Menopause – after the menopause, there is a natural reduction in the level of oestrogen that changes a woman's balance between oestrogen and testosterone. This can lead to androgenetic alopecia.

Low iron stores – tests often show that women with long-term telogen effluvium suffer from low iron stores in the body. This can be measured by having a blood sample analysed for serum ferritin. Although this can be done by your GP, this is a different test to the normal iron tests that measure haemoglobin levels. Research has not established a link between haemoglobin levels and hair loss, but it has shown links between hair loss and low serum ferritin values. In fact, it is not unusual to find you have a normal haemoglobin level but a low serum ferritin reading.

Stress – when an individual experiences intense stress, chemicals in the body will transmit signals to the hair follicles, which causes them to enter a resting phase. During this phase, there is no new hair growth. During the next few months, hair will be shed normally, but new growth will not occur to take its place. This uneven pattern can cause hair to appear thinner and eventually result in hair loss.

Illness – ill health can cause increased hair shedding 10-12 weeks after the start of the problem. The hair loss usually continues for a week or so longer than the time of the illness. Sometimes, additional shedding occurs as a result of the medications given, or if prolonged fever is associated with the illness.

Thyroid imbalances – these affect approximately 2% of younger women and up to 10% of postmenopausal women in the UK and can produce significant changes in hair growth and hair quality. If you suspect a problem, book in with your GP for a blood test.

Natural Support for Hair Loss

To successfully manage hair loss, it's important to try to work out the underlying cause. To do this, it's important to identify possible triggers and have any tests necessary to pinpoint underlying conditions that may be contributing. This will make it easier to choose an appropriate therapy.

Fight Hormonal Hair Loss with Phytoestrogens

One of the most effective ways to tackle hair loss that is related to low oestrogen levels (for example, after the menopause) or excess androgens, is to supplement your diet with phytoestrogens. These natural plant chemicals have a mild oestrogen-like action that can help to keep your hormones functioning in balance. In particular, phytoestrogens are able to sit on hormone receptors in the hair follicles, helping to stop androgens, such as testosterone and DHT, from stimulating hair loss.

The two food types with the highest concentration of phytoestrogens are flax seeds and fermented soya products, such as miso, tempeh and natto. While flax is relatively easy to include dietarily, fermented soya products are not a common feature on most Western menus. For this reason, the easiest way to obtain the benefit of soya is to take a fermented soya supplement.

- Add 1-2 heaped dessertspoons of ground flax seeds to your diet each day
- Supplement with 1000mg of high-potency fermented soya supplement each day that provides 40mg of isoflavones

Lower DHT with Saw Palmetto

Studies have shown that saw palmetto is an effective anti-androgen. Firstly, it lowers levels of DHT in the body by blocking the 5 alpha-reductase enzyme. Secondly, it blocks receptor sites on cell membranes required for cells to respond to DHT. Since DHT is the main factor responsible for androgenetic alopecia, saw palmetto has become a popular remedy for this kind of hair loss.

- Take 1 capsule of a saw palmetto product containing 120-160mg of extract, three times daily with meals

Boost Ferritin Levels

If your health practitioner has done a blood test and confirmed that you have low serum ferritin levels, then addressing your iron levels will help to restore normal hair growth. The best way to do this is to take a combination of an easy-to-absorb form of iron, alongside vitamin C and lysine. This is because lysine and vitamin C are important for the proper absorption of the iron. What's more, studies have shown that this combination of nutrients is more effective at addressing hair loss than using iron supplements alone.

- To optimise iron uptake and hair growth, take the following combination of nutrients three times a day on an empty stomach:
  - 5mg of an easy-to-absorb, bioavailable iron supplement
  - 500mg of the amino acid L-lysine
  - 1000mg vitamin C

Reduce Stress

Since stress is such a common trigger for hair loss, it's a good idea to develop long-term strategies for managing emotional events. More information on this can be found in chapter 17, but if you need a more immediate fix, look for a complex containing the herbs and nutrients below and take two capsules twice a day away from meals.

- **Magnesium** – this mineral is for the enzymes involved in energy metabolism and stress hormone production, but is quickly depleted at times of challenge, often causing fatigue and sleep problems
- **B vitamins** – like magnesium, B vitamins are used up quickly when you're under pressure, but they are key for maintaining a healthy stress response
- **Taurine** – this amino acid supports the production of a neurotransmitter in the brain called GABA, which is responsible for producing feelings of calm and relaxation

- **Theanine** – this is an amino acid found in green tea, which helps to counteract the stimulating effect of caffeine. It can cross the blood-brain barrier and has been found to aid the production of alpha brainwaves, which are associated with "alert relaxation" and general well-being. This nutrient is very good for times of high anxiety
- **Passion flower** – traditionally used to aid relaxation, passion flower also has anti-anxiety effects and can be a useful support during times of stress
- **Lemon balm** – this belongs to a category of herbs called nervines, which nourish the nervous system and support a relaxed state of mind

Take a Hair Support Multi

Whatever the cause of your hair loss, it's important to make sure your body is receiving all the nutrients it needs to grow healthy, luscious hair. The dietary tips in chapter 15 will set you on a firm foundation, but to be sure you're getting adequate levels of everything important for hair growth, it's also advisable to take a hair-specific multi.

- Look for a supplement containing a combination of vitamins C, B6 and B5; biotin, zinc, collagen, GLA, MSM and silicon

Go Natural

Healthy hair relies on a regular delivery of an oily substance called sebum from the hair follicles. Many modern shampoos contain harsh ingredients, such as sodium lauryl sulphate (SLS), that strip these natural oils from the hair, leaving it parched. What's more, SLS and other commercial hair product ingredients have been criticised for their irritating effects on the scalp, leading many people to believe they can contribute to hair loss.

It's interesting to note that we don't actually need to wash our hair with anything at all! Left to it's own devices, regular brushing and the odd rinse with clean water is actually sufficient. The problem is that for hair that has become used to being washed regularly, it can take about four weeks for the natural balance to be restored. In the meantime, you have to live with less than beautiful tresses! A more practical solution is to choose a natural shampoo and conditioner that are SLS-free. These will keep your hair and scalp healthy, as well as looking fabulous.

- Look out for products that have been certified natural by BDIH and which contain pesticide-free plant extracts and natural preservatives. See the resources section at the back of the book for further information

Chapter 14
Cellulite and Veins

Most women take time to care for their upper skin layers, using all kinds of lotions to maintain a healthy, youthful glow, but what about the lower dermal layers, the connective tissues that support the skin and the veins? These also need care and attention, especially when cellulite or vein problems are present.

A Closer Look at the Skin...

Structurally, the skin consists of two parts. The outer, thinner section, composed of layers of epithelial cells, is called the epidermis. This is attached to the inner, thicker, connective tissue layer called the dermis. When talking about cellulite, vascular problems and stretch marks, it is the dermis that is of particular interest.

The dermis is composed of connective tissue containing collagen and elastic fibres and is embedded with blood vessels, nerves, glands and hair follicles. The deeper portion of the dermis is called the reticular region. It consists of dense, irregular connective tissue containing interlacing bundles of collagen and coarse elastic fibres. The spaces between the fibres are occupied by a small number of fat cells, hair follicles, nerves, oil glands and sweat gland ducts.

What is Cellulite?

Cellulite is a term used to describe the dimpled appearance of skin caused by fat deposits that are just below the skin surface. It generally affects the skin on the abdomen, lower limbs and pelvic region, and is thought to affect 80-90% of women once puberty has occurred.

Several factors have been shown to affect the development of cellulite. Changes in the skin 'architecture', alteration of connective tissue structure, genetic factors, diet, lifestyle and inflammatory alterations are all cited. However, the link with puberty suggests that there is a definite hormonal element to the condition, and excess oestrogen has been implicated.

Broken Capillaries

Broken capillaries can appear anywhere on the body, and result when the capillary walls narrow and widen too quickly, causing them to tear. Typically, capillaries that are prone to breaking have reduced strength and elasticity. Common causes of broken capillaries include hot conditions, wind, sunburn, moving from extremes of temperature, physical pressure or actual tissue damage.

Varicose Veins

Varicose veins are veins that have become enlarged and bulging. They develop when the small valves inside the veins stop working properly. In a healthy vein, blood is prevented from flowing backwards by a series of tiny valves that open and close to let blood through. If the valves weaken or are damaged, the blood can flow backwards and can collect in the vein, eventually causing it to be become swollen and enlarged. This can result in tired, aching legs, spider veins, cramps, redness and drying of the area affected, plus poor wound healing.

Stretch Marks

Stretch marks (or striae) are created when the dermis tears. These tears initially appear as red streaks and then gradually fade to a visible silvery line. Stretch marks are usually caused by rapid stretching of the skin during growth, weight gain or a severe force on the skin that is greater than the skin's elasticity. There also appears to be a hormonal link, as stretch marks are more common in puberty, pregnancy and in those on hormonal medical therapies. In addition, glucocorticoid hormones (which include the stress hormone cortisol) can affect the development of stretch marks by preventing fibroblast cells in the skin from forming the collagen and elastin fibres needed for rapid growth.

Supporting Your Skin

There are many ways that you can help to support your skin, through diet, supplements and exercise.

Clean Up Your Diet

It makes perfectly logical sense that a diet rich in antioxidants from fresh fruits and vegetables, high in quality lean protein and rich in essential fatty acids from nuts, seeds and oily fish, is the perfect recipe for skin health.

The key habit to support healthy skin is to include an abundance of different coloured fruits and vegetables on a daily basis to provide your body with a constant supply of beneficial fibre, antioxidants and phytochemicals. It's also important to make sure that you drink your eight glasses of water (or beneficial herbal teas) every day, as this is the only way to make sure toxins are eliminated and the skin is properly hydrated.

Some foods can also exacerbate the appearance of cellulite and vein problems. The worst offenders include alcohol (which dehydrates your body), refined foods (including foods high in artificial additives and sweeteners), fizzy drinks and eating a diet overly high in dairy products and fatty animal meats. In general, following the principles in the hormone-balancing diet (chapter 15) is an excellent starting point. For an extra boost, include a daily green smoothie to increase your fruit and vegetable intake and help remove toxins.

Green Smoothies

Green leafy vegetables are loaded with chlorophyll, which helps us to excrete toxins and reduce excess acidity. They are also an excellent source of protein, as well as bowel-cleansing fibre. By blending greens into smoothies, you maximise their digestibility and, therefore, nutritional value.

To make a green smoothie, simply whizz the greens in a powerful blender (see resources page) with the measured water until puréed and then blend in the fruit for a super-healthy breakfast or afternoon snack. Each recipe makes about a pint of smoothie.

300ml water
25g sunflower seeds (soaked overnight in water)
2 large handfuls of spring greens
1 handful of frozen mango chunks
1 ripe pear

150ml water
150ml apple juice
1 handful of lamb's lettuce
1 head of pak choy
1 banana
1 handful of frozen mixed berries

300ml water
½ bag of spinach
½ an avocado
1 handful of strawberries
1 banana cut into chunks and frozen

300ml water
½ bag of curly kale
4 ripe plums
½ an avocado
1 punnet of blueberries

Tip: You can also add supplements and extra ingredients into green smoothies, such as omega oils, collagen powders, Aloe vera, goji berries and green superfood powders.

Strengthen Connective Tissue

Both the dermis and the blood vessel walls are made up of connective tissue, the strength of which is important for preventing skin and vascular problems. To support these tissues, it's important to make sure your body has a good supply of the building blocks needed to make connective tissue, as well as high levels of the antioxidants needed to keep the collagen and elastin fibres healthy.

Collagen – over time, the connective tissue can become weak as the collagen fibres become damaged and frayed. To keep the skin and blood vessels healthy, these fibres need to be regularly replaced. Although the body is able to do this without assistance, the efficiency of the process depends on having a good supply of necessary raw materials. One way to support this is to take collagen supplements.

Vitamin C – the laying down of new collagen fibres is carried out by an enzyme that requires vitamin C in order to work properly. As an added bonus, vitamin C is also a powerful antioxidant that can help mop up the free radicals that damage collagen fibre in the first place.

- To help keep your skin and blood vessels strong, take a skin-specific collagen drink containing 3630mg hydrolysed collagen, with the supportive action of 55mg each of vitamin C and hyaluronic acid (a natural substance that helps moisturise the skin from within)

Antioxidants – there are also antioxidants that are specifically useful for strengthening blood vessels. These include the flavonoids diosmin and rutin, as well anthocyanidins, which are found in dark berries such as bilberries. These nutrients help scavenge free radicals, strengthen capillaries and veins and reduce inflammation.

- For maximum effect, take 3 capsules a day of a vein-strengthening formula that provides 675mg diosmin, 540mg rutin, 180mg bilberry fruit extract and 15mg vitamin E

Soothe with Aloe

Aloe vera gel can be applied to the skin to soothe and ease tired, dry or poorly conditioned areas. It can also be used to make the skin more taut, which is perfect for areas where cellulite exists.

- For general skin maintenance, apply a high-strength Aloe vera skin gel to the affected area 1-2 times daily

- To support blood vessel health, choose an Aloe gel that also contains vascular-strengthening agents such as vitamins C, E and K, along with horse chestnut, witch hazel, centella asiatica, butcher's broom, arnica, hawthorn, grape seed oil and bilberry

Take up Dry Skin Brushing

Provided your skin isn't sore or broken, dry skin brushing is an excellent way to boost circulation and aid the removal of toxins from the skin. Done on a regular basis (once or twice a day), it can help reduce cellulite and fortify your blood vessels.

How to Dry Skin Brush

Before you start, you'll need to invest in a soft, natural-fibre brush with a long handle. As the name suggests, dry skin brushing should be done on a dry, naked body, preferably just before you have a bath or shower. It's important to brush towards your heart and to use more gentle pressure on delicate areas of skin.

The best technique is to start by brushing the soles of your feet, then work your way up your ankles, calves, thighs and buttocks, brushing vigorously towards your heart. Next, brush your abdomen in a counter-clockwise fashion and, finally, brush from your hands up your arms.

When you've finished brushing, take a warm bath or shower. To optimise your circulation, this should be followed by a cool rinse to stimulate blood flow. Although this sounds like it might leave you feeling cold, it actually helps to send the warm blood to the core of the body, leaving you feeling warm and toasty!

Manage Your Stress

Keep stress to a minimum. As well as glucocorticoids, such as cortisol, influencing development of stretch marks, catecholamines, which are produced by the body in response to stress, have also been linked to an increase in cellulite.

Detox

Many natural health practitioners recommend a regular detox for those who are prone to cellulite, on the basis that excess salt, fatty foods, caffeine and alcohol can all worsen its appearance. This is of benefit to everyone, as it helps you to refocus your diet and might also be useful for addressing any hormonal imbalances that may be affecting your skin and other areas of your health. But for a liver detox to be truly effective, it's also important that your digestive system is working efficiently, so it can properly excrete any toxins your liver releases. To find out more about detoxifying these systems, read chapter 2.

Quit Smoking

Research studies conclusively state that smoking reduces the elasticity of the skin, as well as depleting the levels of important skin-supporting antioxidants, such as vitamin C.

Exercise

Exercise increases circulation, which carries vital nutrients to the lower levels of the skin and helps to remove waste products. In addition, exercise keeps weight down (reducing chances of stretch marks occurring) and also helps reduce cellulite by toning muscles near the surface of the skin.

One particularly beneficial form of exercise for boosting skin and vascular health is rebounding. Put simply – performing small controlled exercises while bouncing on a mini trampoline! It helps to improve circulation, increase the capacity of the heart and lungs, reduce stress and tension and improve muscle tone. It also boosts the flow of the lymphatic system, which helps to remove toxins from the skin. If you're new to rebounding, it's best to start with just 10 minutes a day and gradually build up. There are also various fitness DVDs available to help you get the best out of your regime.

Chapter 15
Hormone Balancing – Dietary Factors

When it comes to hormones, a balanced diet means more than just managing to get your 'five-a-day'! A few simple changes can have very positive effects.

Amazing Vegetables

We're all being encouraged to eat our five-a-day, though strictly speaking, nutritionists would encourage you to eat more than that, as well as urging you to include a wide variety of plant foods. This is because including a variety of different colours of fruit and vegetables helps to ensure you get a good intake of lots of different kinds of antioxidants.

In addition to antioxidant properties, certain vegetables are also rich in constituents that could help hormonal balance and make an excellent addition to a hormone-balancing diet.

- Indole-3-carbinols – these compounds, found in cruciferous vegetables such as cabbage, Brussels sprouts, cauliflower, spring greens and broccoli, help to transform dangerous oestrogen into more benign forms. They have also been shown to stop the growth of breast cancer cells by inhibiting the action of a specific enzyme
- Apigenin – there is evidence that a plant chemical called apigenin can inhibit aromatase, the enzyme that converts androgens to oestrogens. Good sources of this flavone include celery, bell peppers, parsley, chamomile and peppermint
- Isoflavones – the isoflavones found in fermented soya products have also been shown to be potent aromatase inhibitors. For more information, see the section below on phytoestrogens

Increase Your Fibre

We know, from reading about how oestrogen is metabolised in chapter 2, that the digestive system and, in particular, a slow gut transit time, can greatly influence hormonal status. Fibre intakes are known to help the 'clearance' of oestrogen breakdown products from the body, thus preventing reabsorption, which can cause oestrogen levels in the body to rise.

Increasing dietary fibre is easy. Eat more fruits and vegetables (wash them well, and leave the skin on when possible) and also think about including cold milled or sprouted ground flax seeds in your diet, which are high in fibre and also contain good levels of omega 3 fatty acids. Sprinkle them on cereals or salads, add to smoothies or stir into sauces.

Balance Your Blood Sugar

In chapter 3, we read about the importance of balancing blood sugar and how this can be achieved by eating a low-glycaemic diet. But what does this really mean in practice?

Go Low-GI

The glycaemic index (or GI) of a food is a measure of the speed at which sugars are released from the food into the bloodstream, compared to pure glucose. It is a scientific way of assessing the potential impact of sweet and starchy foods on our blood sugar levels. Low-GI foods release their sugars slowly, having a minimal impact on blood sugar levels, while high-GI foods are those that are most likely to create a 'sugar rush'.

To support good blood sugar balance, the majority of the starchy foods in your diet should be low-GI foods. This means choosing wholegrains and pulses, and in addition, avoiding high-GI foods, such as sweets and white processed foods.

The table below outlines the glycaemic index of some common foods. In general, you should focus on eating foods from the low-GI column, include some from the moderate-GI column and limit high-GI foods to special occasions.

Low-Glycaemic	**Moderate-Glycaemic**	**High-Glycaemic**
Apple juice	Kiwi	Watermelon
Cherries	Mango	Banana
Oranges	Peaches	Grapes
Plums	Pineapple	Melon
Apples		Dried fruit
Pears		
Dried apricots		
Grapefruit		
Stewed fruit (no sugar)		
Berries		

Low-Glycaemic	Moderate-Glycaemic	High-Glycaemic
Chocolate (70% cocoa solids)*	Honey	Sugar
	Other Chocolates	
Tomato or vegetable juice	Fruit squash (diluted)	Alcohol Fizzy drinks
Rye bread	White basmati rice	White rice
Brown rice	Buckwheat	Biscuits
Wholewheat pasta	Pastry	Rice cakes
Barley	White pasta	Cornflakes
Whole oats	Potato crisps	Wheat cereals
Oatcakes	Sugar-free Muesli	White bread
Quinoa	Wholemeal bread Rye crackers Popcorn (fresh, no sugar coating	French bread Corn chips
Baked beans	Kidney beans	Broad beans
Chickpeas		
Butter beans		
Lentils		
Sweet potato	Sweetcorn	Parsnips
Nuts and seeds	Carrots (raw) Peas Boiled potatoes (skin on)	Carrots (cooked) Baked potato Chips Cooked beetroot
Milk (skimmed/whole)	Ice cream*	
Yoghurt (plain)		

* Not an excuse to eat regularly!!

Eating Protein Regularly

A regular intake of protein can also aid blood sugar balance. This is because protein slows down how fast the sugar is released from sweet and starchy foods. The best protein choices are: skinless organic chicken or turkey, fish, organic eggs, live low-fat natural yoghurt, raw nuts, seeds, quinoa, beans, lentils, tofu, tempeh, goat's cheese and cottage cheese.

Getting a Good Balance

To make sure you have a good balance on your plate, aim for one palm-sized portion of low-GI starch, one palm-sized portion of lean protein and three handfuls or more of different coloured vegetables at each main meal. If you're having beans and pulses, these are half starch and half protein, so go for two palm-sized servings rather than combining them with extra starch.

Eat Good Fats

With many women's hormonal conditions, essential fatty acids can play a part, either in helping to manage knock-on symptoms, such as poor skin and lack-lustre hair, or aiding directly by rebalancing prostaglandin levels to help deal with symptoms such as painful periods.

Omega 3 oils, from fish oil or flax seed oil, are most useful, though you might like to take a combination of omega 3 and 6 oils together. This will give you a great platform on which to have hormonal balance (see each chapter for specific information about condition-related use of essential fatty acids).

Don't forget, you can also increase your intake of omega fats from dietary sources by eating two portions of oily fish (salmon, mackerel, sardines, trout etc) each week and including food such as omega-3-enriched eggs, avocados, cold pressed flax seed oil, cold pressed hemp seed oil, nuts and seeds, as well as nut and seed butters. Interestingly enough, B vitamins, which are also important for hormone production and clearance from the body, are also found in nuts, seeds and eggs!

Include Phytoestrogens

We've already seen in the previous chapters that phytoestrogens can be useful in the management of specific female health problems, but they can also be a great dietary addition for general hormone balancing. Phytoestrogens are simply plant chemicals that have a mild oestrogen-like action. They are incredibly effective for helping with both low and high oestrogen levels and, in that respect, we can call them oestrogen-balancing.

If body levels of natural, highly biochemically active oestrogens are low, then soya isoflavones can lock into oestrogen receptors in the body, contributing some oestrogenic action. If natural oestrogen levels in the body are too high, soya isoflavones can lock into oestrogen receptors, giving weakly oestrogenic action (thus downregulating oestrogenic action in the body).

The table below lists some of the most important dietary sources of phytoestrogens:

Phytoestrogens food sources	Phytoestrogens content (μg/100g)	Phytoestrogens food sources	Phytoestrogens content (μg/100g)
Flax seeds	379380.0	Mung bean sprouts	495.1
Soya beans	103920.0	Dried apricots	444.5
Tofu	27150.1	Alfalfa sprouts	441.4
Soy yoghurt	10275.0	Dried dates	329.5
Sesame seeds	8008.1	Sunflower seeds	216.0
Flax bread	7540.0	Chestnuts	210.2
Multigrain bread	4798.7	Olive oil	180.7
Soy milk	2957.2	Almonds	131.1
Hummus	993.0	Green beans	105.8
Garlic	603.6	Onion	32.0

Note: Although soya beans are high in phytoestrogens, these are only effective once they have been activated by fermentation. This means tempeh, miso and natto are better choices than soya milks or tofu, which can be difficult to digest. Since these fermented traditional soya foods are less widely available in the West, a good alternative is a wholefood, fermented soya supplement that provides 40mg of soy isoflavones per tablet.

Eat More Methionine

Methionine is important for liver function, particularly through its ability to detoxify oestrogen, so ensuring a good intake is an excellent aid to hormonal balance. Foods which are high in methionine include trout, cod, tuna, mackerel, sardines, turkey, lean steak, yoghurt, eggs, cottage cheese, Brazil nuts, sesame seeds, tahini, sunflower seeds, pumpkin seeds, soya (fermented forms preferred, such as miso, tempeh, natto and soya yoghurt), beans, pulses, onion and garlic.

Keep a Healthy Weight

Throughout the book, we have seen that carrying excess body weight can result in hormonal imbalances, while severe weight loss can result in low oestrogen activity, compromised thyroid function and raised cortisol levels. All of these can lead to a reduction, or cessation, of ovulation.

Excess weight can result in excess androgens and oestrogen in the body (and reduce levels of progesterone). It can also influence the levels of follicle-stimulating hormone and prolactin, which, in turn, influence menstrual regularity and the ability to ovulate.

The good news is that hormones tend to return to normal when excess weight is lost. This can be achieved by following the dietary guidelines above (or in the chapter relating to your specific condition), monitoring your portion sizes and doing some kind of exercise for at least 30 minutes, five times a week.

A Little Extra Help

There's no escaping the fact that weight loss requires commitment to a sensible diet and exercise programme! However, certain supplements can help to make it easier to stick your diet or ensure you get the best out of your efforts by helping you to burn fat more effectively.

- PI2 Inhibitors – this revolutionary extract from potato helps manage appetite and hunger naturally. It works by enhancing the release of the body's own satiety factor, CCK. Clinical studies have shown that taking one capsule, an hour before your two largest meals, can increase feelings of fullness, aid portion control, curb snacking and accelerate weight loss!

- HCA – this natural extract from the tamarind fruit can aid weight loss by blocking one of the enzymes that converts excess sugars into fat and by activating the biochemical pathways that burn fat for energy. A good dose is one to two 450mg tablets 30 minutes before a meal, up to three times a day

- CLA – when used in combination with a regular exercise programme, CLA can increase fat loss and help in reshaping problem areas of the body, such as the hips and thighs. A good dose is three 1000mg capsules per day

Keep Your Thyroid Healthy

Thyroid balance is important when considering hormonal health, as we know that thyroid conditions can influence the menstrual cycle and, also, the ability to ovulate.

One of the most important minerals for the thyroid is iodine, the main dietary sources of which are fish, seafood and sea vegetables. One of the richest supplies can be found in the seaweed kelp, a very tough and leathery seaweed that is usually taken in tablet form due to its poor palatability. A good dose to take is two 300mg tablets per day.

Another option is to include more sea vegetables in your diet. Some health food shops also stock culinary seaweeds, either in fresh or dried form, which can be added to salads, soups and stews, while products such as nori sheets can be used to make sushi or can be lightly toasted for a crunchy snack. For an extra boost, you can also buy dried kelp sheets to add to stews and soups during cooking – just remember to remove them before serving!

Cut Out Caffeine

You might feel like you need your 'kick-start' caffeine in the morning, and also, mid-afternoon, late afternoon and with your evening meal, but have you considered the impact of caffeine on hormonal health? From a holistic perspective, caffeine places an extra burden on liver function. While it is active, it's also a central nervous system stimulant. As a result, there are a number of known side effects, including thirst, anxiety, irritability, mood swings, depression, insomnia, fast heart rate, flushing, hyperglycaemia, muscular tremors, diarrhoea, increased urination, stomach ache, dizziness and many more!

Drinks and foods high in caffeine	Great alternatives
Coffee Tea Cola drinks Energy drinks Chocolate (including hot chocolate) Anything containing guarana Green tea	Filtered/bottled water Lemon juice in hot water – great for the liver Herbal teas Fruit teas Rooibos (Redbush) tea – high in antioxidants and tastes similar to traditional 'black' tea Water-processed decaffeinated coffee Dandelion coffee Grain coffees e.g. barley or chicory based coffee alternatives

A word of warning – if you decide to give up caffeine completely, it's likely that you'll experience some withdrawal symptoms. These include headaches, muscle aches or stiffness, difficulty concentrating and irritability. The good news is that these symptoms only last about five days, after which you'll feel amazing! Some people prefer to go 'cold turkey' and get the withdrawal out the way. For others, gradually reducing their intake of caffeine or swapping it for lower caffeine options, such as green tea, is more favourable.

Reduce Alcohol

Alcohol most definitely has an impact on hormonal balance, as can be seen in conditions where excess alcohol has lead to compromised liver function. Compromised liver function leads to compromised oestrogen clearance, which could contribute to many conditions linked with oestrogen excess. If your hormonal imbalance is pronounced, it would be wise to cut alcohol completely from your diet. If you feel you must drink (if perhaps you feel it helps you to relax, helping to cut stress, which influences hormonal balance also), then only have one or two small glasses a week.

Avoid Xenoestrogens

As well as women's own internal oestrogen production, xenoestrogens from the environment can also influence hormonal balance. Found in certain commercially raised non-organic meat, pesticides, plastics, fuels and medications, xenoestrogens are substances that bind to an oestrogen receptor, altering the function of the endocrine system and causing adverse health effects. They are usually synthetic chemicals and are, therefore, an extra biochemical challenge for the body to break down. This can lead to an increase in oestrogen 'load' in the body over time.

Environmentalists have previously highlighted how xenoestrogens have made their way into our ecosystems, causing reproductive disruption in both animals and men, not to mention the hormonal imbalance that can be experienced by women exposed to these hormone-disrupting compounds. Although complete avoidance isn't practical, it's a good idea to try and reduce your exposure to key sources of xenoestrogens.

Look out for....

- Commercially raised meat and dairy
- Pesticides and herbicides
- Plastics and plastic food wraps
- Polystyrene cups
- Garden chemicals and wood treatments
- Car exhausts and indoor toxins
- Birth control pills
- Air fresheners and perfumes
- Paints, lacquers and solvents
- Commercial sunscreens
- Toiletries that contain parabens
- Food additives

Note: Packaging made of PET does not contain bisphenol A – the major xenoestrogen in other plastics.

Tips for avoiding xenoestrogens:

- Use glass or ceramics whenever possible to store food and water
- Heat up your food using a glass or ceramic bowl covered with a dish – when plastic is heated, it diffuses very rapidly into food
- Use a simple detergent with less chemicals
- Use natural toiletries without parabens – see resources page
- Use natural pest control, not pesticides, e.g. a weak solution of grapefruit seed extract
- Avoid synthetic chemicals as much as possible
- Don't use herbicides – a 20:80 solution of vinegar and water may be sprayed on weeds instead
- Buy hormone-free/organic meats and dairy products
- Buy organic produce grown without pesticides, herbicides, synthetic fertiliser
- Use condoms without spermicide for birth control instead of birth control pills

Chapter 16
Healthy Lifestyle, Healthy Hormones

The pace of life for many women is incredibly hectic, with hardly any time at all to stop and think about the impact of everything on hormonal health. What should we change?

Stress

All along, in the chapters of this book, we have read over and over again, how stress impacts on hormonal balance; - not just sex hormones, but other hormones too such as those involved in blood sugar balance and metabolism. But stress affects us in simpler ways too:

1. Stress causes the body to use up key hormone balancing vitamins and minerals more quickly. This is particularly true for B vitamins, magnesium and zinc.
2. Stress often leads to much less healthy eating. We simply can't be bothered to cook fresh or fancy food, and that often leads to poor intakes of the vitamins and minerals essential for hormonal balance.
3. Stress often causes digestive upset. Digestive health is essential for oestrogen balance, as it's involved in helping to clear it from the body. It's also important for proper nutrient uptake.
4. Stress can make us take on unhelpful lifestyle patterns, such as smoking or excess alcohol which robs the body of essential protective factors such as antioxidants.

For these reasons, it's essential to find ways of managing stress. This might simply be sitting in the garden with a cup of herbal tea or having a night out with friends. Alternatively you might like to look over Dr Mark's chapter (chapter 17) to find out more about the mind-body tools that can be helpful for managing stress and negative emotions.

Whichever route you choose to manage your stress, there are also a number of supplements and herbs that you can consider to support your body and a more relaxed frame of mind.

- B-vitamins are essential, not only in hormone making and breakdown processes, but also for the biochemical pathways used during stress. In addition to this, people who are stressed often don't eat properly, which can result in poor dietary intake of the B-vitamins. To ensure you're getting enough during times of stress, consider taking two to three tablets of a good B-complex with 15-25mg daily of vitamins B1, B2, B3 and B6 and around 50mg of B5 daily. For extra support, look for a formulation that contains around 200mg of vitamin C per tablet and 50 mg of Siberian ginseng as this herb really supports hectic lifestyles.
- Many of the processes involved in energy production and stress hormone manufacture rely on a good supply of magnesium. Unfortunately, chronic stress depletes magnesium levels, which can worsen fatigue and interfere with sleep. To counteract this, take the equivalent of 400-800mg of an easy-to-absorb form of magnesium in the evening to offset stress-induced depletion and aid restful sleep.
- The mineral zinc is also a consideration as studies show stress can deplete zinc levels quickly. In ideal dose is 20mg per day, but ensure you pick a formula that also contains a balanced amount of copper.
- Rhodiola is a herb traditionally used for the relief of symptoms associated with stress, such as fatigue and exhaustion. It also helps increase mental performance and decrease cortisol response to stress. This makes it ideal for times when you feel 'tired but wired', have lots of commitments to juggle or are trying to meet a deadline. The recommended dose is one tablet containing 200mg of rhodiola rosea extract per day.

Don't Smoke

Quitting smoking is one of the most beneficial things you can do for your overall health as well as for your hormonal balance. Whilst smoking might seem to provide a way to relieve stress, it actually increases the release of adrenal hormones such as cortisol (a stress hormone) and androgens (male hormones). This can, in turn, upset blood sugar levels and interfere with sex hormone balance.

Smoking is also very toxic to the body, because it greatly increases the levels of highly reactive chemicals called free radicals. Left unchecked these cause oxidative damage, which is associated with chronic health problems and accelerated ageing. This extra free radical load also puts additional pressure on the body's antioxidant defences, so much so that research studies from America have suggested that all smokers need to take 200mg of vitamin C daily, just to prevent vitamin C deficiency!

When it comes to actually giving up, there are lots of different options available and a huge number of resources. There are charities that provide online and telephone support and many healthcare centres have staff specially trained to help people give up smoking. There are also alternative therapies such as hypnosis, which can help. With so many choices out there, it's a good idea to do some research to work out which approach it going to work best for you. Further information can be found in the resources section at the back of the book.

Increase Your Exercise

Study after study has shown that exercise positively influences brain chemistry, increasing the release of feel-good chemicals in the brain as well as helping us to release pent-up tension and angst! But it also has more basic, physiological benefits. For example in inflammatory conditions (think of painful periods, polycystic ovaries, fibroids), physical movement can ease inflammation and associated symptoms such as fluid retention, swelling, and dull nagging aches. Exercise also increases blood flow to all areas of the body, which can help speed up detoxification and increase the delivery of vital nutrients.

To get these benefits, you need to exercise regularly. This means doing something active for 30 minutes or more everyday. This might be structured exercise such as going to the gym, swimming or going to an exercise class, or more lifestyle – based activity such as briskly walking to the shops or climbing stairs. The key is variety – don't just stick to one type of exercise, which could overwork a particular area instead mix and match cardiovascular exercise (the sort that makes you out of breath) with strength training. Muscles take time to recover so it's best to leave at least 48 hours between resistance training sessions.

It's also important to choose the kind of exercise you do carefully. Strenuous high-intensity exercise can activate the body's stress response (which can have knock on effects on your hormones), as well as increasing free radical load. So it's important not to overdo it and take things at your own pace, working with your body, rather than against it! Below is a list of some different types of beneficial exercise.

- Brisk walking – This is easy to fit in around everyday life and doesn't require any special equipment.
- Stair climbing – Aim for three session of 10 minutes each day.
- Dancing – Join a class or simply dance energetically to your favourite tunes. Belly dancing is particularly good for getting your feminine energy flowing and boosting blood flow to the reproductive organs!

- Swimming – Good for cardiovascular health as well as toning.
- Aqua classes – Brilliant fun and the added resistance of the water helps to build muscle.
- Rebounding – Fantastic for stimulating detoxification and circulation as well as for aiding weight loss.
- Yoga/Pilates – Excellent for improving muscle strength, flexibility and posture
- Weight Training – This is an excellent way to build muscle and improve body composition (more muscle = less fat!). Ask a gym instructor or personal trainer to set you up with some exercises to do in the gym or join a weight-training-based exercise class.
- Boxercise/Combat Aerobics – Based on fighting moves, these classes are great for releasing pent-up anger and keeping in shape.

Chapter 17
How to Manage Your Emotions
by Dr Mark Atkinson

Our emotions, for better or for worse, are always influencing our health, mood and decisions that we make. In this chapter, I am going to reveal some really simple ways to manage your emotions, in a way that will support the nutritional recommendations made by Holly, as well as help you improve your health and make you happier.

What are Emotions?

The starting point for working with our emotions is to understand that emotions are simply information. They are messages telling you about what is happening in your body and mind and whether you are meeting their needs. For optimum health, your body needs to have healthy food, rest, sleep, relaxation, physical activity, water, warmth and shelter and it needs to be relatively free from a variety of body-related problems, such as imbalances of hormones, neurotransmitters (chemicals that communicate mood) and nutrients, as well as allergies, inflammation and toxicity. If these needs aren't being met, your body will communicate it to you through distressing emotions, such as irritability and sadness.

You also have emotional needs, which include the need for security, giving and receiving positive attention, connection with the wider community, an intimate, close relationship with at least one other person, autonomy, status, competence, privacy, meaning and purpose. If these aren't being met, your emotions will tell you. For example, if I am not meeting my need for friendship, I might experience sadness or loneliness; if I feel threatened by someone and therefore feel unsafe, I might feel anger and fear; and if don't feel competent in what I do, I might experience embarrassment, fear and nervousness. By listening to your emotions, you will often discover an unmet need, which, when met, will result in the emotion disappearing. Once the emotion has served its function, it no longer needs to be there.

Women and Emotions

In our society, women are often regarded as being more emotional than men. However, research has found that men and women actually experience very similar levels of emotion; it's just that women are more likely to show that emotion. This is partly due to social conditioning. As a woman, you are much more likely to be exposed to emotionally focused conversations and encouraged to express your emotions verbally, although for most women, the exception is the expression of anger. When compared with men, women[1]:

- express their emotions more easily and are less likely to exert control over what they feel
- are more likely to share their emotions with others
- express their emotions with more intensity
- use more emotive language
- are more likely to have their behaviour affected by emotions
- are less likely to express emotions relating to control, such as pride, anger and jealousy
- are more likely to remember details of an emotionally charged event or experience and experience greater emotional intensity in response to those memories
- are likely to experience mood swings because of fluctuations in their hormone levels – for example, up to 60% of women will experience mood swings prior to their period, mainly due to changes in hormones and levels of the brain neurotransmitters serotonin and noradrenaline

In a nutshell, women tend to be influenced and affected by their emotions more than men, but they also have the ability to deal with this more effectively than men!

When Emotions Become a Problem

Emotions become a problem when we sedate, control or deny them. At the heart of this is the tendency to divide emotions into two groups; positive and negative, and then further subdivide them: joy, happiness and peace (positive); and anger, rage, sadness and fear (negative). This polarisation of emotions is unfortunate, because they all contribute to being 'real' and the experience of being human. Negating any of these blunts our ability to experience the full spectrum of emotions, which, in turn, disconnects us from a valuable source of insight and information. Emotions are therefore not inherently bad. Anger is not bad, rage is not bad and sadness is not bad; what determines whether they are healthy or unhealthy is our relationship to them. Below are the five main 'relationships' we have with our emotions:

1. Feeling them fully, accepting them as they are without wanting to do anything with them and allowing them to pass through and out of your awareness – healthy
2. Discharging them, through physical activity or sharing your thoughts – healthy
3. Allowing them to overwhelm you and acting them out – unhealthy
4. Suppressing or consciously resisting them, which often involves distracting yourself or chemically changing the way you feel through behaviours such as eating, drinking alcohol or smoking – unhealthy
5. Repressing them; in other words, they are automatically prevented from coming up in the awareness – very unhealthy

In my own work, I've found that people who suppress and repress their emotions the most are so-called 'nice' people. However, by adopting a 'nice all the time' approach in order to avoid conflict and receive positive attention from others, true feelings of anger, sadness and resentment – all of which are normal and natural – get bottled up. Doing this increases the likelihood of emotionally induced illness, such as chronic pain and irritable bowel syndrome. Getting in touch with your emotions, feeling them fully and being authentic and honest is, for me, at the heart of emotional health.

Top Six Tips for Managing Emotions

1. Anytime you are feeling stressed or overwhelmed – breathe

I teach my patients 4/7 breathing. As it states, you breathe in to the count of four, then breathe out to the count of seven. Repeat a couple of times and notice how much better you feel. As you do this, adjust your posture – relax your shoulders, look up slightly and allow yourself to smile. What's great about 4/7 breathing is that it takes you out of the whirlwind of your emotions and into a much calmer, more grounded state of mind.

2. Ask yourself: What do I need to do to bring my body-mind into balance?

Behind most of your emotions, and certainly stress, is an unmet emotional or physical need, which I discussed earlier on. For example, you might be experiencing stress and tension because your blood sugar has dropped too low, or because you are sleep deprived or because you need some rest. At another time, you may experience stress because you are resisting reality, haven't spoken your truth; or maybe you have a tendency towards perfectionism and have set yourself an impossible deadline. So, having calmed yourself with 4/7 breathing (or using whatever else works for you), ask the question above and then allow yourself to receive an answer. What is the underlying unmet emotional and/ or physical need being communicated to you through this emotion you are feeling? In my experience, the top needs behind the emotion are:

- The need to stop fighting reality
- The need to speak your truth
- The need to express/process your emotions
- The need to eat, sleep or rest
- The need to make a decision or take positive practical action

Having identified the underling need (this takes practice), if practical, take an action to meet that need. For example, have something to eat, rest for a moment, or call a friend to share what is on your mind. Having done so, notice how the stress dissipates. Once you get the message, the body-mind no longer needs to create stress.

3. Stop sedating and controlling your emotions

In order to get in touch with your emotions so that you can relate to and work with them in a more healthy way, one of the first – and potentially, very challenging – tasks is to illuminate the ways in which you sedate, control and avoid and distract yourself from your emotions. These behaviours include excessive busyness, caretaking, overeating, compulsive judging of others and oneself, excessive control, manipulation, lying, using food and sugar to change the way we feel, drinking alcohol, people-pleasing, overachieving, gossiping, excessive television watching, addictions, comparing, overthinking, avoiding intimacy and overworking. Take some time to identify and write down your own emotional avoidance behaviours. From now on, anytime you notice yourself using one of these strategies, smile to yourself and say silently: 'oh, there is my emotional avoidance strategy'. If it's appropriate, use one of the healthy emotional management strategies below.

4. Use EmoTrance

EmoTrance is the number one tool I teach my patients for managing their emotions in a healthy way. EmoTrance is based on the idea that a healthy state of mind and body arises when subtle energy (chi) flows without interruption through and out of the body. When we hold on to, or suppress or repress, an emotional upset, this stops the energy from flowing, which, in turn, leads to distressing mental, and sometimes physical, symptoms. EmoTrance is designed to restore the flow of energy.

How to Use EmoTrance

The following exercise will provide you with an experiential taste of EmoTrance. I would suggest giving yourself at least 20 minutes to do this, at a time when you know you won't be disturbed.

1. Think of a statement, fact, thought or criticism that causes you to feel upset or to feel 'negative' emotions. This could be a person or a phrase that upsets you, such as 'you're fat', 'you're useless', or 'you disappoint me'.

2. Write this issue down on a piece of paper, turn it face down, take a deep breath, then turn it back over and allow yourself to feel any emotions. If you don't feel anything, choose another issue.

3. Pay close attention to where you feel it in your body. If there is more than one site, choose the one that feels strongest. What you are feeling is just trapped energy or emotion that wants to move.

4. If you can, gently place your hands on that area and get a sense of the direction in which the energy wants to go. If you don't get an immediate indication, start massaging the area with your hands, holding the intention of softening it as you do so.

5. When the energy starts to move, which it will do, get a feel for which part of your body it wants to exit through. This can be any location – top of the head, mouth, nose, hands, feet – anything goes! If it's not obvious which exit route it wants to take, just be patient and continue softening until it starts exiting your body.

6. Allow all the energy to exit your body. If it appears to get stuck, gently rub that area or trace the route you feel it wants to take with one of your hands as that often helps.

7. More often than not, there will be residual energy in your body, so to make sure that all of the emotional charge has been deactivated, repeat the whole procedure again, starting from number 3.

8. Keep repeating until you feel no unpleasant sensation at all. On average, it takes two to three cycles. If you feel lighter, more energised and much clearer around the issue, then you have successfully deactivated that emotional trauma – well done!

9. Take a moment to consider how this experience will change your behaviour and the way you feel about the issue.

Using this tool might at first appear to be a bit tricky; but, once you've tried it a couple of times, you'll see how straightforward it is. The key is to be patient with yourself. Part of your mind will try to rush you and convince you that it isn't working for you. If this happens to you, just slow down, breathe deeply and continue.

In summary, when you have an emotionally-charged issue to work with:

- Locate where you are feeling the energy
- Tell it to 'soften and flow'
- Get a sense of where it wants to exit your body
- Allow it to flow and, if you catch yourself trying to force it, or getting frustrated by it, breathe deeply and let go
- Repeat until you have gone as far as you can

I recommend you use EmoTrance both reactively – in the moment you get emotionally triggered – and also proactively. For example, check in with yourself at the end of the day and ask yourself whether you are carrying any left over emotions from the day. If so, release them using EmoTrance. I also recommend writing down a long list of upsets from the past and using EmoTrance on each of these. One a day is usually enough. This process of letting go of the past can be very healing and liberating work.

5. Consider other healthy ways of managing your emotions

In addition to using EmoTrance, you might also want to consider:

Sharing

One of the simplest ways to process your emotions is to share what you are feeling with someone who is present, accepting of your reality and able to listen to you, with the intention of truly hearing what you have to say. To find someone who can do this is a rarity – however, most people have at least one person they know. If not, and especially if you have any significant emotional or mental health challenge, you could work with a good counsellor.

Support Groups

There are many self-help support groups for women with specific health challenges. In addition to being part of network of women going through similar challenges, they can be a source of good information. Here are some of the main groups:

PMS	www.pms.org.uk
PCOS	www.verity-pcos.org.uk
Endometriosis	www.endometriosis-uk.org
Fibroids	www.fibroidnetworkonline.com
Infertility	www.fertilityfriends.co.uk

Keeping a Journal

Writing down your stressful thoughts and worries and journaling about stressful events can really help to offload and process the emotions that you are experiencing. For more information, I recommend the book Writing to Heal by Dr Pennebaker.

6. Develop a relaxation practice

Learning how to relax is an essential part of living a healthy, balanced life. Regular relaxation can help you manage stress, reduce levels of pain and discomfort, increase wound healing and even help you to access greater creativity[2]. Here are some suggestions to get you started:

- Build a relaxation period into your daily routine. I recommend between fifteen and thirty minutes each day
- Choose a couple of relaxation practices and try them out to discover which works for you. They include, among others, meditation, prayer, yoga, chi kung, walking in nature, massage, taking a hot bath, listening to music, progressive muscle relaxation, mantras, self-hypnosis and guided imagery
- Mindfulness meditation is a skill and practice that is increasingly recognised as an effective way to reduce pain, relieve stress, decrease addictive cravings, increase self-awareness, reduce hot flushes and enhance emotional intelligence[3]. Mindfulness is a way of paying attention to, and seeing clearly, whatever is going on in your life. While being mindful, you are bringing an attitude of openness, curiosity and acceptance to the reality of whatever it is you are noticing. You might not like or want whatever is happening to happen, but you are welcoming the reality of it. For information on books and CDs, see the resources page

References

1. Hutson-Comeaux S, Kelly J. Gender stereotypes of emotional reactions: how we judge an emotion as valid. *Sex Roles: A Journal of Research*. July 2002.
2. Benson, H. *The Relaxation Response.* Morrow; 1976.
3. Teasdale, J D et al. Prevention of Relapse/Recurrence in Major Depression by Mindfulness-Based Cognitive Therapy. *Journal of Consulting and Clinical Psychology*. 2000; 68(4):615–23.

Resources

Supplements and Omega Excellence Cold Pressed Oils, Butters and Seeds

Higher Nature Ltd
Website: www.highernature.co.uk
Tel: 0800 458 4747

High-Powered Blenders and Juicers

UK Juicers Limited
Unit 5 Harrier Court
Airfield Business Park
Elvington
York
YO41 4EA
Website: www.ukjuicers.com
Tel: 01904 757070

Juiceland Ltd
Unit 2 Bradman Complex
Bradman Road
Knowsley Industrial Park
Liverpool
L33 7UR
Tel: 0151 549 2190
Website: www.juiceland.co.uk

Gluten and Dairy Free Recipe Books

Cooking Without by Barbara Cousins

Cooking Without Made Easy
by Barbara Cousins

Vegetarian Cooking Without
by Barbara Cousins

Gluten, Wheat and Dairy Free Cookbook
by Antoinette Savill

The AiA Gluten and Dairy Free Cookbook
by Marilyn Le Breton

The Allergy-Free Cookbook
by Michelle Berriedale-Johnson

The Wheat and Dairy Free Cookbook
by Terence Stamp and Elizabeth Buxton

Skin Care Guide

Nutritional Solutions for Optimising Skin Health
Available through Higher Nature Ltd
Website: www.highernature.co.uk
Tel: 0800 458 4747

Natural Skin and Hair Care

The Energys Range
Available through Higher Nature Ltd
Website: www.energysskincare.com
Tel: 0800 458 4747

Quitting Smoking

Quit – UK charity that helps people give up smoking

Helpline: 0800 00 22 00
Email counseling:
stopsmoking@quit.org.uk
Website: www.quit.org.uk

NHS Stop Smoking Service
Helpline: 0800 022 4332
Website: www.smokefree.nhs.uk

Mindfulness Meditation CDs

'*Guided Meditations: For Calmness, Awareness and Love*' by Bodhipaska

'*Guided Mindfulness Meditation*' by Jon Kabat-Zinn

Trauma Therapies

The rewind technique:
www.hgi.org.uk/register/

EMDR: www.emdrassociation.org.uk

Somatic experiencing:
www.traumahealing.com

Nutrition and Natural Health

Nutrition Solutions for Optimising Digestive Health

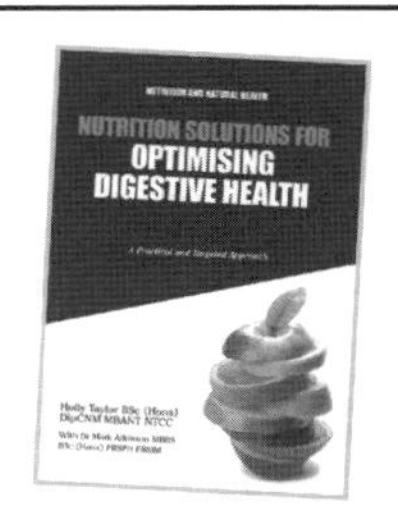

Holly Taylor BSc (Hons) DipCNM MBANT NTCC

With Dr Mark Atkinson MBBS BSc (Hons) FRSPH FBSIM

Packed with practical advice, this book provides all the information you need to build a personalised plan for optimal digestive health. Whether you suffer from heartburn or IBS, constipation or Candida, this book has the answers!

Starting with a top-to-bottom tour of the digestive system and a fascinating insight into the fate of a sandwich, this book goes on to cover a whole range of common digestive disorders, with expert guidance on nutrition and natural therapies.

It offers:

- Advice on transforming your eating habits for life-long digestive health
- Key symptom analysis for fast identification of individual problem areas
- Tools to identify digestive imbalances and food sensitivities
- Effective action plans to optimise digestive health and heal the gut
- Essential information about rebalancing intestinal ecology
- Top tips for managing stress and emotional digestive triggers

RRP £4.99

For more information or to order, please email anothercountrypublishing@gmail.com.

Nutrition and Natural Health

Trim Track Plan

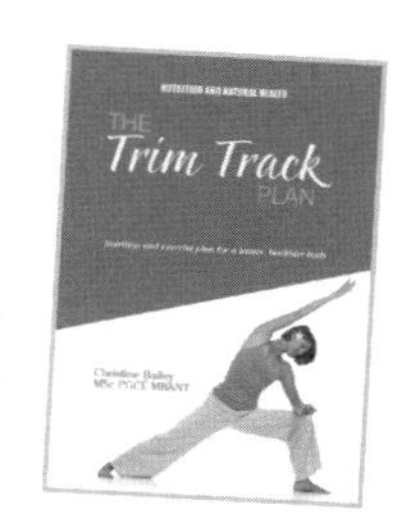

Christine Bailey MSc PGCE MBANT Nutritionist (BSc Hons)

The Trim Track Plan is much more than just about losing weight. It is designed to help you improve body composition, increase muscle mass and develop a lean, toned body. The Plan will help reshape your body for optimal health and enable you to adopt healthier habits to positively improve your long-term health.

RRP £3.99

For more information or to order, please email anothercountrypublishing@gmail.com.

Nutrition and Natural Health

Intelligent Way to Lose Weight

Christine Bailey MSc PGCE MBANT Nutritionist (BSc Hons)
With Dr Mark Atkinson MBBS BSc (Hons) FRSPH FBSIM

Are you confused by all of the conflicting advice on diets and nutritional health? Have you tried dieting, but failed to keep your weight off? Does food, and/or the thought of food, dominate your life? Would you like to know how to permanently lose weight, put a stop to cravings, and feel much better about yourself?

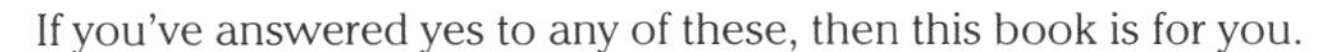

If you've answered yes to any of these, then this book is for you.

Dr Mark Atkinson, integrated medical doctor and expert in healthy weight loss, will share with you his personalised holistic programme for losing inches from your waist and maximising your health, wellbeing and mood. Unlike most diet plans, which advocate just changing the types and amounts of foods that you eat in order to lose weight, *The Intelligent Way to Lose Weight* does this, plus shows you how to identify and resolve the five most common barriers to easy and permanent weight loss. Furthermore, you will learn how to:

- Make food choices that are suited to your metabolism
- Overcome emotional eating
- Increase your energy and lift your mood
- Get in tune with your body's wisdom
- Permanently dissolve food cravings
- Transform your body image and confidence

RRP £7.99

For more information or to order, please email anothercountrypublishing@gmail.com.

Colloidal Silver

Zoe Adams

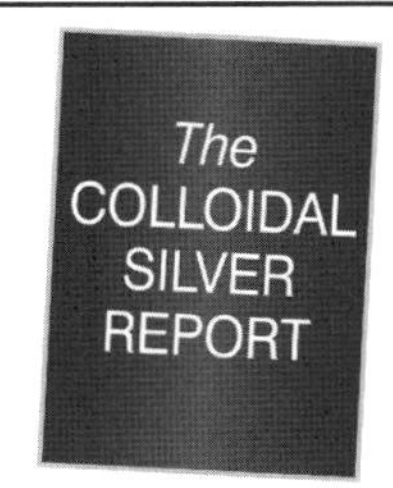

Everything you need to know about colloidal silver - a versatile antiseptic and antimicrobial spray containing 10ppm silver with a multitude of uses all described in depth, together with a description of exactly how and why it is so effective.

RRP £2.50

For more information or to order, please email anothercountrypublishing@gmail.com.